Enabling Novel Treatments for Nervous System Disorders by Improving Methods for Traversing the Blood–Brain Barrier

PROCEEDINGS OF A WORKSHOP

Lisa Bain, Noam I. Keren, and Clare Stroud, *Rapporteurs*

Forum on Neuroscience and
Nervous System Disorders

Board on Health Sciences Policy

Health and Medicine Division

The National Academies of
SCIENCES · ENGINEERING · MEDICINE

THE NATIONAL ACADEMIES PRESS
Washington, DC
www.nap.edu

D1247558

THE NATIONAL ACADEMIES PRESS 500 Fifth Street, NW Washington, DC 20001

This activity was supported by contracts between the National Academy of Sciences and the Alzheimer's Association; Brain Canada Foundation; Cohen Veterans Bioscience; the Department of Health and Human Services' Food and Drug Administration (5R13FD005362-02) and National Institutes of Health (NIH) (HHSN26300089 [Under Master Base #DHHS-10002880]) through the National Center for Complementary and Integrative Health, National Eye Institute, National Institute of Mental Health, National Institute of Neurological Disorders and Stroke, National Institute on Aging, National Institute on Alcohol Abuse and Alcoholism, National Institute on Drug Abuse, and NIH Blueprint for Neuroscience Research; Department of Veterans Affairs (VA240-14-C-0057); Eli Lilly and Company; Foundation for the National Institutes of Health; Gatsby Charitable Foundation; George and Anne Ryan Institute for Neuroscience at The University of Rhode Island; Janssen Research & Development, LLC; Lundbeck Research USA; Merck Research Laboratories; The Michael J. Fox Foundation for Parkinson's Research; National Multiple Sclerosis Society; National Science Foundation (BCS-1064270); One Mind; Pfizer Inc.; Pharmaceutical Product Development, LLC; Sanofi; Society for Neuroscience; and Takeda Development Center Americas, Inc. Any opinions, findings, conclusions, or recommendations expressed in this publication do not necessarily reflect the views of any organization or agency that provided support for this project.

International Standard Book Number-13: 978-0-309-47307-1
International Standard Book Number-10: 0-309-47307-1
Digital Object Identifier: https://doi.org/10.17226/25044

Additional copies of this publication are available for sale from the National Academies Press, 500 Fifth Street, NW, Keck 360, Washington, DC 20001; (800) 624-6242 or (202) 334-3313; http://www.nap.edu.

Cover image courtesy of Dr. Viviana Gradinaru, California Institute of Technology, Pasadena, California.

Suggested citation: National Academies of Sciences, Engineering, and Medicine. 2018. *Enabling novel treatments for nervous system disorders by improving methods for traversing the blood–brain barrier: Proceedings of a workshop.* Washington, DC: The National Academies Press. doi: https://doi.org/10.17226/25044

The National Academies of
SCIENCES · ENGINEERING · MEDICINE

The **National Academy of Sciences** was established in 1863 by an Act of Congress, signed by President Lincoln, as a private, nongovernmental institution to advise the nation on issues related to science and technology. Members are elected by their peers for outstanding contributions to research. Dr. Marcia McNutt is president.

The **National Academy of Engineering** was established in 1964 under the charter of the National Academy of Sciences to bring the practices of engineering to advising the nation. Members are elected by their peers for extraordinary contributions to engineering. Dr. C. D. Mote, Jr., is president.

The **National Academy of Medicine** (formerly the Institute of Medicine) was established in 1970 under the charter of the National Academy of Sciences to advise the nation on medical and health issues. Members are elected by their peers for distinguished contributions to medicine and health. Dr. Victor J. Dzau is president.

The three Academies work together as the **National Academies of Sciences, Engineering, and Medicine** to provide independent, objective analysis and advice to the nation and conduct other activities to solve complex problems and inform public policy decisions. The National Academies also encourage education and research, recognize outstanding contributions to knowledge, and increase public understanding in matters of science, engineering, and medicine.

Learn more about the National Academies of Sciences, Engineering, and Medicine at **www.nationalacademies.org**.

PLANNING COMMITTEE ON ENABLING NOVEL TREATMENTS FOR NERVOUS SYSTEM DISORDERS BY IMPROVING METHODS FOR TRAVERSING THE BLOOD–BRAIN BARRIER[1]

HUSSEINI MANJI (*Co-Chair*), Janssen Research & Development, LLC
DANICA STANIMIROVIC (*Co-Chair*), National Research Council of Canada
FRANCESCA BOSETTI, National Institute of Neurological Disorders and Stroke
E. ANTONIO CHIOCCA, Harvard Medical School
VIVIANA GRADINARU, California Institute of Technology
CHENGHUA GU, Harvard Medical School
JAMES KOENIG, National Institute of Neurological Disorders and Stroke
SARAH H. LISANBY, National Institute of Mental Health
ROGER LITTLE, National Institute on Drug Abuse
WILLIAM PARDRIDGE, University of California, Los Angeles
STEVEN PAUL, Voyager Therapeutics, Inc.
ERIC SCHAEFFER, Janssen Research & Development, LLC
AJAY VERMA, United Neuroscience

Health and Medicine Division Staff

CLARE STROUD, Forum Director
SHEENA M. POSEY NORRIS, Program Officer
NOAM I. KEREN, Associate Program Officer
DANIEL FLYNN, Research Assistant
ANDREW M. POPE, Director, Board on Health Sciences Policy

---

[1]The National Academies of Sciences, Engineering, and Medicine's planning committees are solely responsible for organizing the workshop, identifying topics, and choosing speakers. The responsibility for the published Proceedings of a Workshop rests with the workshop rapporteurs and the institution.

FORUM ON NEUROSCIENCE AND NERVOUS SYSTEM DISORDERS[1]

STEVEN HYMAN (*Chair*), Broad Institute of Massachusetts Institute of Technology and Harvard University
STORY LANDIS (*Vice Chair*), Director Emeritus, National Institute of Neurological Disorders and Stroke
SUSAN AMARA, Society for Neuroscience
RITA BALICE-GORDON, Sanofi
KATJA BROSE, Chan Zuckerberg Initiative
EMERY BROWN, Harvard Medical School and Massachusetts Institute of Technology
JOSEPH BUXBAUM, Icahn School of Medicine at Mount Sinai
SARAH CADDICK, Gatsby Charitable Foundation
ROSA CANET-AVILES, Foundation for the National Institutes of Health
MARIA CARRILLO, Alzheimer's Association
E. ANTONIO CHIOCCA, Harvard Medical School
TIMOTHY COETZEE, National Multiple Sclerosis Society
JONATHAN COHEN, Princeton University
FAY LOMAX COOK, National Science Foundation
JAMES DESHLER, National Science Foundation
BILLY DUNN, Food and Drug Administration
MICHAEL EGAN, Merck Research Laboratories
JOSHUA GORDON, National Institute of Mental Health
HANK GREELY, Stanford University
RAQUEL GUR, University of Pennsylvania
MAGALI HAAS, Cohen Veterans Bioscience
RAMONA HICKS, One Mind
RICHARD HODES, National Institute on Aging
STUART HOFFMAN, Department of Veterans Affairs
MICHAEL IRIZARRY, Eli Lilly and Company
INEZ JABALPURWALA, Brain Canada Foundation
FRANCES JENSEN, University of Pennsylvania
GEORGE KOOB, National Institute on Alcohol Abuse and Alcoholism

---

[1]The National Academies of Sciences, Engineering, and Medicine's forums and roundtables do not issue, review, or approve individual documents. The responsibility for the published Proceedings of a Workshop rests with the workshop rapporteurs and the institution.

WALTER KOROSHETZ, National Institute of Neurological Disorders and Stroke
JOHN KRYSTAL, Yale University
ALAN LESHNER, American Association for the Advancement of Science (Emeritus)
HUSSEINI MANJI, Janssen Research & Development, LLC
DAVID MICHELSON, Merck Research Laboratories (until December 2017)
JAMES OLDS, National Science Foundation (until December 2017)
ATUL PANDE, Tal Medical
STEVEN PAUL, Voyager Therapeutics, Inc.
STEPHEN PEROUTKA, Pharmaceutical Product Development, LLC
RODERIC PETTIGREW, National Institute of Biomedical Imaging and Bioengineering (until November 2017)
EMILIANGELO RATTI, Takeda Pharmaceuticals International
TAREK SAMAD, Pfizer Inc.
DOUGLAS SHEELEY, National Institute of Dental and Craniofacial Research
TODD SHERER, The Michael J. Fox Foundation for Parkinson's Research
DAVID SHURTLEFF, National Center for Complementary and Integrative Health
PAUL SIEVING, National Eye Institute
NORA VOLKOW, National Institute on Drug Abuse
ANDREW WELCHMAN, Wellcome Trust
DOUG WILLIAMSON, Lundbeck
STEVIN ZORN, MindImmune Therapeutics, Inc.

Health and Medicine Staff

CLARE STROUD, Forum Director
SHEENA M. POSEY NORRIS, Program Officer
NOAM I. KEREN, Associate Program Officer
DANIEL FLYNN, Research Assistant
JIM BANIHASHEMI, Financial Officer (until October 2017)
BARDIA MASSOUDKHAN, Financial Associate (from October 2017)
ANDREW M. POPE, Director, Board on Health Sciences Policy

Reviewers

This Proceedings of a Workshop was reviewed in draft form by individuals chosen for their diverse perspectives and technical expertise. The purpose of this independent review is to provide candid and critical comments that will assist the National Academies of Sciences, Engineering, and Medicine in making each published proceedings as sound as possible and to ensure that it meets the institutional standards for quality, objectivity, evidence, and responsiveness to the charge. The review comments and draft manuscript remain confidential to protect the integrity of the process.

We thank the following individuals for their review of this proceedings:

CHOI-FONG CHO, Brigham and Women's Hospital
AGNES V. KLEIN, Health Canada
ELISA E. KONOFAGOU, Columbia University
SARAH H. LISANBY, National Institute of Mental Health
BERND STOWASSER, Sanofi
AJAY VERMA, United Neuroscience, Inc.

Although the reviewers listed above provided many constructive comments and suggestions, they were not asked to endorse the content of the proceedings nor did they see the final draft before its release. The review of this proceedings was overseen by **LESLIE Z. BENET,** University of California, San Francisco. He was responsible for making certain that an independent examination of this proceedings was carried out in accordance with standards of the National Academies and that all review comments were carefully considered. Responsibility for the final content rests entirely with the rapporteurs and the National Academies.

Contents

Applying the Consortia Model to BBB Research, 36
Final Thoughts, 39

APPENDIXES

1

Introduction and Overview[1]

Despite substantial advances in developing treatments for the serious illnesses that affect people worldwide, there remains a tremendous unmet need in the treatment of complex neurological diseases, including neuropsychiatric and neurodegenerative disorders, said Husseini Manji, global therapeutic head for neuroscience at Janssen Research & Development. Chief among the challenges that have hindered the development of therapeutics for central nervous system (CNS) disorders is the blood–brain barrier (BBB), he said.

The BBB has been historically viewed simply as a physical barrier, according to Danica Stanimirovic, director of the Translational Bioscience Department at the National Research Council of Canada. Yet we now know that it is a complex dynamic system that involves multiple cell types and transporters and interacts with other elements in its environment, she said. Stanimirovic added that exploiting this new evolving understanding of the BBB could enable the development of more intelligent drug-delivery strategies. Manji agreed, noting that new tools and technologies that would allow molecules to cross the BBB could enable treatment with a range of large molecules, including antibodies and other biologic agents (biologics).

The BBB has stymied CNS treatment development and relegated it to orphan status, said Steven Hyman, director of the Stanley Center for

[1]The planning committee's role was limited to planning the workshop, and this Proceedings of a Workshop was prepared by the workshop rapporteurs as a factual summary of what occurred at the workshop. Statements, recommendations, and opinions expressed are those of individual presenters and participants, and have not been endorsed or verified by the Health and Medicine Division (HMD) of the National Academies of Sciences, Engineering, and Medicine, and they should not be construed as reflecting any group consensus.

Psychiatric Research at the Broad Institute of Harvard and Massachusetts Institute of Technology. Manji suggested that the field is now at an inflection point and poised to move forward in developing technologies to traverse the BBB. To galvanize the scientific community to take on this challenge and bring different resources to bear, the Forum on Neuroscience and Nervous System Disorders of the Health and Medicine Division of the National Academies of Sciences, Engineering, and Medicine convened a workshop on September 8, 2017. The workshop planning committee was tasked with bringing together experts from academia, government, the biotechnology and pharmaceutical industries, disease-focused organizations, nonprofit foundations, and other interested stakeholders to explore current and evolving strategies for traversing the BBB to deliver therapeutics to the CNS (see Box 1-1). Workshop participants also discussed gaps to address, including potential regulatory obstacles, and explored strategies for accelerating research and clinical translation through the establishment of consortia and public–private partnerships (PPPs). This workshop explored mechanisms that are relevant across conditions, but it did not delve deeply into any specific condition.

The committee will develop the agenda for the workshop, select and invite speakers and discussants, and moderate the discussions. A summary of the presentations and discussions at the workshop will be prepared by a designated rapporteur in accordance with institutional guidelines.

BOX 1-1
Statement of Task

An ad hoc committee will plan and conduct a 1-day public workshop that will bring together key stakeholders from government, academia, industry, and disease-focused organizations to explore the current development of novel methods for traversing the blood–brain barrier to deliver therapeutics for nervous system disorders and identify potential opportunities for moving the field forward.

- Provide an overview of current knowledge on the role of the blood–brain barrier biology and delivery mechanisms, examining gaps in our current knowledge that future research may address.
- Discuss brain–blood barrier passive and active mechanisms that challenge development and delivery of effective therapeutic interventions to central nervous system targets.
- Highlight current data and innovative approaches for delivery of therapeutics across the brain–blood barrier harnessing such meth-

ods as chemical modifications, Trojan horse approaches, physical targeting and disruption, nanoparticles, ultrasound, and other technologies.

- Explore potential opportunities for catalyzing development of novel treatments that cross the blood–brain barrier—from the preclinical to clinical phase—with an emphasis on risks, levers, and potential collaborative efforts among sectors.

WORKSHOP OBJECTIVES

The workshop was designed to explore the challenges associated with the BBB that have thus far stymied development of CNS drugs, examine new technologies that could address these challenges, and highlight potential opportunities for moving the field forward.

ORGANIZATION OF THE PROCEEDINGS

The following proceedings summarize the workshop presentations and discussions. Chapter 2 briefly summarizes the structure and function of the BBB, diseases related to its breakdown, challenges that arise in designing therapeutics that will cross or bypass the BBB, and opportunities to address these challenges. Chapter 3 surveys the modalities and technologies currently in development for traversing the BBB to deliver therapeutic molecules to the CNS, as well as models being used to facilitate the discovery and development of new drugs to treat CNS diseases. Chapter 4 explores regulatory issues and concerns for investigators to consider as they move through preclinical and clinical phases of development.

Chapter 5 examines innovative funding models and partnership strategies to accelerate research and facilitate clinical translation of these technologies by increasing collaboration and establishing PPPs across various stakeholder communities, including academia, industry, the private sector, and federal agencies.

2

Traversing the Blood–Brain Barrier: Challenges and Opportunities

The workshop focused on strategies for delivering drugs to the brain by crossing or bypassing the blood–brain barrier (BBB). Many of the approaches currently in development target neurodegenerative diseases, such as Alzheimer's disease (AD). However, the pursuit of treatments for orphan indications, such as mucopolysaccharidosis types 1 and 2, may be more tenable as they may benefit from the Food and Drug Administration's (FDA's) Accelerated Approval Pathway, suggested Francesca Bosetti, program director for Stroke in the Neural Environment Cluster at the National Institute of Neurological Diseases and Stroke. In addition, individuals affected by rare serious diseases may be more motivated to participate in clinical trials. Hyman added that techniques for traversing or circumventing the BBB may also be applied effectively to psychiatric disorders, such as mood disorders and schizophrenia. Since these conditions could require speedier delivery of drugs to the brain as well as shorter-term persistence of the drug in the brain, different technologies and approaches may be needed, he said.

HOW THE BBB PRESENTS
CHALLENGES FOR DRUG DELIVERY

The BBB is a continuous endothelial membrane that, along with pericytes and other components of the neurovascular unit, limits the entry of toxins, pathogens, and blood cells to the brain, said Berislav Zlokovic, director of the Zilkha Neurogenetic Institute at the Keck School of Medicine, University of Southern California (Zlokovic, 2011). It accomplishes this through the actions of numerous transport systems. However, it also represents an obstacle to central nervous system (CNS) drug delivery, said

Zlokovic. Moreover, he said, the fact that blood vessel patterns tightly follow brain circuits suggests that the vascular system, and therefore the BBB, plays an important role in normal brain function, aging, and disease.

Breakdown of the BBB is associated with several neurodegenerative disorders, such as AD, amyotrophic lateral sclerosis (ALS), Parkinson's disease (PD), multiple sclerosis, and chronic traumatic encephalopathy, as well as stroke and infectious diseases of the brain, such as those caused by the human immunodeficiency virus, said Zlokovic. He added that there are also rare monogenic neurological diseases associated with genetic defects in nonneuronal cells that cause disruption of the neurovascular unit and breakdown of the BBB (Zhao et al., 2015). Some of these diseases are associated with a change in expression of transporters. For example, Zlokovic and colleagues have shown that reduced expression of glucose transporter 1 (GLUT1), which mediates glucose transport into the brain, is associated with neuronal dysfunction and degeneration in AD (Winkler et al., 2015). The question is whether these disease-associated gene alterations that are associated with BBB breakdown contribute to the disease or are innocent bystanders, said Zlokovic. While the workshop focused on mechanisms to enable delivery of drugs to the brain by crossing or bypassing the BBB, Zlokovic noted that a pathologically disrupted BBB is unhealthy, and that healthy blood vessels will be needed to deliver drugs to the brain. His laboratory has thus explored approaches to prevent disruptions of the BBB that may contribute to disease. In AD, for example, the pathogenic protein amyloid-beta (Aβ) interacts with a receptor for advanced glycation end products (RAGE), disrupting the BBB and enabling the transport of Aβ across the BBB, said Zlokovic. RAGE blockers are currently being tested in phase III trials to see if they can suppress the accumulation of Aβ in the brain (Deane et al., 2003). Zlokovic and colleagues are also investigating the mechanisms by which an enzyme called activated protein C (APC) may protect neurons by tightening the BBB (Griffin et al., 2015). A variant of APC called 3K3A-APC, which optimizes the cell-signaling properties of the enzyme (Griffin et al., 2016), is currently in phase II trials for stroke, said Zlokovic.

There have been many attempts over the past 25 years to develop biologics for brain diseases, said William Pardridge, professor of medicine at the University of California, Los Angeles. These include attempts to deliver neurotrophins to treat ALS and PD, and growth factors to treat stroke. The earliest efforts delivered the drugs by subcutaneous injection, not appreciating that they would not cross the BBB. In stroke, the BBB is disrupted but not until 12 to 24 hours after the event, long past the "window of opportunity" for neuroprotection, said Pardridge. Subsequent efforts tried injections directly into the brain or through a technique called convection-enhanced diffusion. Although these studies showed that drug levels in the cerebrospinal fluid (CSF) exceeded those in the plasma, these trials were nevertheless unsuccessful, indicating that CSF levels do not reflect BBB penetration, said Pardridge. More recently, investigators have begun to exploit specialized transport systems in the microvasculature as a means of delivering drugs across the BBB, he said. These are the focus of this workshop.

OVERVIEW OF CHALLENGES

During the workshop presentations and discussions, participants identified gaps and challenges associated with development of methods for traversing the BBB and to improve therapeutic delivery to the nervous system. The issues listed here, and attributed to the individuals who made them, are expanded on in succeeding chapters.

Understanding the Complex Biology of the BBB

The major reasons for the high attrition rates in CNS drugs include a limited understanding of drug permeability at the BBB, drug distribution in the brain, and target engagement in the brain, said Danica Stanimirovic. Understanding the BBB molecular makeup should enable identification of new targets for both managing disease and delivering drugs, she said. However, Robert Thorne, assistant professor in pharmaceutical sciences at the University of Wisconsin–Madison, called the study of the BBB an "orphan field," which lacks the appreciation and funding it is due within the neuroscience community.

Zlokovic described the complex interplay of cells and molecules that shape BBB structure and function, including not only endothelial cells, pericytes, and vascular mural cells but also microglia and astrocytes, and molecules such as various BBB junction proteins, transporters, receptors, and ion channels (Zhao et al., 2015). Regional heterogeneity of these components adds further complexity to understanding structure and function, said Zlokovic.

The complex biology of the BBB contributes to the difficulty in studying many aspects of BBB disruption, including the role of circadian rhythms and differences between wakefulness and sleep states, said Thorne, and the timing of its disruption during stroke, said Pardridge.

Understanding Drug Delivery and Distribution in the Nervous System

According to Thorne, attempts to deliver drugs systemically to the brain have not been fully translated to the clinic, in part because delivering drugs intended for the brain via systemic routes may result in unacceptably high levels in the periphery. Even direct infusions into the brain or CSF have had limited success, he said, in part because diffusion of large molecules, such as enzymes, from the CSF to the brain is limited. Other delivery approaches may be more promising, such as delivery to perivascular spaces—the fluid- and connective tissue–filled areas surrounding blood vessels in the subarachnoid space between the brain and the skull, said Thorne. However, achieving efficient drug delivery will require better characterization of the precise distribution of molecules in the CNS using different strategies, and a better understanding of how molecules move in the CSF and perivascular spaces, he said. In addition, he cited the need to examine other variables that may influence distribution of molecules in the CNS, including body position, intracranial pressure, effects of various diseases, and individual variations.

Viral delivery of drugs presents other challenges, said Viviana Gradinaru, Heritage principal investigator at the California Institute of Technology. Most work has been done with adenoassociated viruses, although these have a small packaging capability. There are also challenges with regard to region and cross-species specificity, she said. Also not well understood are the mechanisms underlying the use of focused ultrasound to facilitate drug delivery, said Alexandra Golby of Brigham and Women's Hospital.

Creating Suitable Models for Understanding BBB Dysfunction

Zlokovic commented that available methods in humans to study BBB dysfunction do not distinguish among the different mechanisms of permeability, for instance paracellular via transcytosis versus transcellular via breakdown of tight junctions. While animal models can distinguish among these mechanisms, they present other challenges, he said. For example, anatomical and size differences between species affect both how a molecule crosses the BBB and whether it hits its desired target, said Douglas

Hunt, head of regulatory affairs for ArmaGen. Larger species also have more complex brains, said Stanimirovic. Differences in the availability of transporters and receptors, for example, can result in selective efficacy of biologics and antibodies, she said. Pharmacokinetic and pharmacodynamic studies may also not translate well between small and large animals, said Balu Chakravarthy, senior research officer at the National Research Council of Canada.

Despite the limitations of animal models, they are essential to develop potential biomarkers and to gather strong efficacy data before undertaking expensive preclinical studies and even more expensive clinical studies, said Bosetti.

Conducting Complex Preclinical Studies

The preclinical evaluation of complex molecules capable of traversing the BBB is not simple, but it is necessary to understand the attributes that would enable them to be moved through the development process into clinical translation, said Stanimirovic. Evaluating the toxicity of complex fusion molecules delivered to the brain presents multiple challenges, including immunogenicity, targeting of different brain areas, and the potential for cross-linking with surface proteins and evoking a cascade of high-level immune activation, known as a "cytokine storm," said Matthew Whittaker, a pharmacology and toxicology reviewer at FDA.[1] He added that even when drugs are designed to target the brain, systemic toxicity needs to be evaluated. Species-specific biologies add to the complexity not only in terms of toxicity but also in terms of efficacy, because different species may express different levels of a desired target receptor, said Hunt. He added that to evaluate dosing in preclinical studies, predictive models would be advantageous.

Addressing Barriers to Translation into Effective Treatments

Translational challenges include a lack of preclinical outcomes that mimic clinical outcomes and inadequate biomarkers, said Stanimirovic. Among existing biomarkers, CSF biomarkers that show a drug is getting into the brain may not correlate with improved clinical function, said Hunt. This raises ethical concerns about doing lumbar puncture in children, he

---

[1] The discussion represents the views of the participants and should not be construed to represent FDA's views or policies.

said. For orphan indications, key challenges include defining appropriate clinical end points and meeting enrollment goals, particularly in light of the heterogeneity of many of these conditions, said Hunt.

To accelerate translation, Stanimirovic also suggested a need to streamline regulatory pathways while managing toxicity, safety, and immunogenicity. Deepa Rao of FDA's Division of Psychiatry Products noted that this can be particularly challenging when therapeutics combine multiple components, such as a drug and device, two enzymes, or an antibody and enzyme. Hunt added that determining the risk–benefit ratio for molecules that target the brain may be more complex than for drugs targeting other organ systems.

Streamlining Siloed Research Programs and Attracting Scientists to the Field

Progress in understanding the BBB and developing technologies to traverse it are also hindered by the manner in which research is conducted. For example, Frank Walsh, founder and chief executive officer of Ossianix, said that pharmaceutical companies operate in silos, such as pharmacology and toxicology, rather than integrating efforts toward a common goal. Pharmaceutical companies have also failed to appreciate the importance of delivery science, said Thorne.

Shortcomings in academia also contribute to slow progress in the BBB field, especially in its historical failure to attract and train a sufficient number of scientists to the field, said Thorne. Many academic neuroscience programs still overlook the cerebrovasculature and CNS barriers in their training even today, in part because they lack qualified faculty with appropriate expertise in CNS barriers science and vascular biology. Even if a pharmaceutical company wanted to resource a BBB program, it would find few trained scientists to hire, he said. Edmund Talley, program director of channels, synapses, and circuits at the National Institute of Neurological Diseases and Stroke, added that academia has underappreciated regulatory science.

OVERVIEW OF POTENTIAL OPPORTUNITIES

Stanimirovic said that it is time to address the evolving concept of the BBB as a very dynamic fluid membrane that expresses many different transporters, shuttles, and pores; and that interacts very closely with other elements of the environment, including glia, pericytes, neurons, and microglia. Only then can this new evolving knowledge of the BBB be exploited for developing new and more targeted drug-delivery approaches that combine novel molecules with innovative delivery strategies, she said.

Developing and Refining Novel Approaches for Drug Delivery

Innovation is now on the drug delivery side, said Pardridge. Proteins and polypeptides may now be delivered to the brain through a variety of approaches:

- Trojan horse approaches using fusion molecules (Walsh)
- Exploiting the inflammatory response by using macrophages and monocytes to transport therapeutic molecules (Kabanov)
- Using viral vectors to transport genes into the brain (Gradinaru)
- Disrupting the BBB with focused ultrasound to enable delivery of therapeutic molecules (Golby)
- Bypassing the BBB by delivering drugs to the brain intranasally, via the olfactory or trigeminal nerve pathways (Thorne)

Developing New Models That Better Represent the BBB

Translation of basic science to clinical applications is a complex process that will require increased development of both in vitro and animal models, said Stanimirovic.

- In vitro models have played a significant role in facilitating the discovery and development of new drugs for CNS diseases, said Choi-Fong Cho, a neuroscientist at Brigham and Women's Hospital and Harvard Medical School. A spheroid model developed in her lab enables high-throughput drug screening.
- Stem cell technologies have enabled the development of 2-D and 3-D models to study BBB permeability and transport (Zlokovic).
- More than 40 animal models have been developed to study BBB breakdown in human disease and to tease out mechanisms that contribute to it, such as pericyte degeneration and fibrinogen deposition (Zlokovic).
- Systems biology approaches using mathematical modeling can help elucidate mechanisms and predict responses in terms of both safety and efficacy (Shah).

Developing Biomarkers

The field is increasingly moving toward the preclinical use of biomarkers of target engagement and toxicity, said Stanimirovic.

- Biomarkers could improve the efficiency of clinical trials, thus lowering their cost (Patel).
- Biomarkers that confirm drug delivery into the brain and BBB permeability status would enable subject stratification for clinical trials (Bosetti).
- Novel imaging and molecular techniques also provide opportunities to study brain vasculature and BBB disruption in living animals and humans, and correlate these with cognitive changes (Zlokovic).

Building Collaborations to Advance Understanding of the BBB

Because the BBB is complex and truly multidisciplinary, collaborative and cooperative research approaches are essential, said Stanimirovic. Bernd Stowasser, head of global public–private partnerships at Sanofi, and a core member of the European Federation of Pharmaceutical Industries and Associations (EFPIA) Innovative Medicines Strategy Priority Workgroup, added that collaborations such as public–private partnerships provide benefits for all stakeholders: academic researchers, industry, and patients.

- Because the BBB occupies a unique interface between the vasculature and the brain, it may provide the opportunity for research dollars to have a substantial effect (Thorne).
- Advancing innovative BBB research will require an increased focus on basic and translational science, attracting more young researchers to the field, and supporting them to stay in the field (Brose, Gu, Lisanby, Talley, Thorne).
- Consortia could develop training programs and incentives to encourage scientists to enter and remain in the field (Thorne).
- Attracting the interest and expertise of investigators from outlying fields would encourage innovation in BBB science (Campany).

3

Modalities and Technologies for Brain Delivery

Highlights

- Three biologics have been approved by the Food and Drug Administration (FDA) for central nervous system diseases, but all of them require direct injection into the cerebrospinal fluid surrounding the brain and spinal cord (Thorne).
- Therapeutic agents can be delivered to the brain by either crossing or bypassing the blood–brain barrier (BBB) through a variety of approaches (Schaeffer).
- The Trojan horse approach shuttles a therapeutic agent into the brain by fusing the therapeutic molecule to a molecule that engages a receptor on vascular endothelial cells, thus initiating receptor-mediated transcytosis (Boado, Chakravarthy, Walsh).
- Immune cells such as monocytes and macrophages, which are capable of infiltrating the brain in the presence of inflammation, may also be used to ferry therapeutic molecules and have been used successfully in mouse models to deliver neurotrophic factors and enzymes (Kabanov).
- Microbubbles created during the delivery of focused ultrasound may be able to carry therapeutic molecules into the brain (Golby).
- Since the nasal mucosa is highly vascularized, therapeutics delivered intranasally may access the brain via the olfactory and trigeminal nerve pathways, thus bypassing the BBB (Thorne).
- Multicellular spheroids can be used as an in vitro platform for screening molecules to determine if they cross the BBB (Cho).
- A mathematical model has shown promise as a means to predict delivery of therapeutics to the brain and appropriate dosing (Shah).

NOTE: These points were made by the individual speakers identified above; they are not intended to reflect a consensus among workshop participants.

The bottleneck in effectively treating neurological and neurodegenerative diseases has been in delivery of drugs to the central nervous system (CNS), said Robert Thorne. There are currently three approved biologics that are delivered into the brain or spinal cord, he said. These are ziconotide, a peptide derived from a cone snail toxin that acts on calcium channels to relieve pain; nusinersen, an antisense oligonucleotide to treat infantile spinal muscular atrophy; and cerliponase alfa, an enzyme-replacement therapy for Batten disease, a rare inherited CNS disorder in children. All of these therapeutics are administered directly into the cerebrospinal fluid (CSF) either by injecting them directly into the lumbosacral subarachnoid space or into the ventricular space in the brain. By better understanding how these biologics are working, improvements may be possible that increase their effectiveness and better facilitate their delivery, said Thorne. Billions of dollars have also been spent on trials of immunotherapy drugs delivered systemically, but these trials have yielded disappointing results so far, said Thorne. Thus, he said the field is starting to appreciate that perhaps these antibodies are not reaching their appropriate targets within the CNS and that alternative delivery routes need to be explored further. Andrew Welchman of Wellcome concurred, noting that it is not enough to say that a treatment does not work—you have to know why. Quantifying how well the therapeutics have been delivered is thus very important but not well understood.

Delivering therapeutic agents to the brain by crossing the blood–brain barrier (BBB) can be accomplished in several different ways, according to Eric Schaeffer of Janssen Research & Development. One of the most active areas in industry uses "Trojan horses" (Pardridge, 2006) to ferry cargo across the brain capillary endothelium by engaging receptors on the endothelial cell surface, such as the transferrin or insulin receptor, according to Schaeffer. Viruses have also devised ways to cross the BBB, and thus they provide a powerful means of delivering therapeutic molecules to the brain, said Schaeffer. The BBB can also be temporarily disrupted with externally applied stimulation, such as ultrasound, he said. Finally, he described an approach that bypasses the BBB by delivering molecules intranasally or intrathecally. Developing any of these approaches into effective therapies for brain diseases will require technological advances in several areas, including the development of in vitro high-throughput screening assays, said Schaeffer. These approaches for traversing the BBB to deliver therapeutics to the CNS are addressed in more detail in the next sections.

CROSSING THE BBB

Several methods and technologies are being studied and implemented to deliver drugs across the BBB. Some methods exploit innate biological mechanisms in the BBB, while others employ external disruption or engineered transport of therapeutics.

The Trojan Horse Approach

According to Frank Walsh, the characteristics required of the shuttle in the Trojan horse approach include rapid uptake and efficient transfer of the cargo into the brain tissue, potency in therapeutic doses, ability to work with different types of cargo (such as antibodies or enzymes), safety, and translatability across rodent and human species. Many different transporters are in development as shuttles, including the transferrin receptor, the insulin receptor, and the low-density lipoprotein receptor-related protein 1 (LRP-1), said Walsh. These receptors enable transport of cargo to the brain tissue via a process called receptor-mediated transcytosis (Jones and Shusta, 2007). Through genetic engineering, antibodies or peptides that bind to these receptors are linked to the therapeutic molecule of interest, creating a fusion molecule capable of rapid brain uptake and delivery of the therapeutic molecule. Walsh's company, Ossianix, for example, isolated cross-species binders to the transferrin receptor from synthetic libraries derived from primordial single-domain shark antibodies. These anti-transferrin receptor 1 variable new antigen receptors (anti-TfR1 VNARs) provided rapid, robust, and prolonged uptake into the brain tissue and neurons at therapeutic doses, said Walsh. As shown in Figure 3-1, this fusion protein bound to the monoclonal antibody rituximab enabled high, rapid transfer of the drug to the brain, as well as persistence for as long as 6 days. Balu Chakravarthy presented data from preclinical studies done with another compound that uses the Trojan horse approach. This therapeutic agent, KAL-ABP-BBB, comprises three components (see Figure 3-2): the "Trojan," an antibody called FC5, which was derived from camelid and engages the receptor-mediated transcytosis process; an antibody fragment (Fc) that enhances serum half-life; and a therapeutic molecule called amyloid binding peptide (ABP), which is designed to bind to and clear amyloid.

Chakravarthy and colleagues first demonstrated that the fusion molecule is transported across the BBB in vitro. This was followed by studies in mice, which showed that the drug is transferred to the brain in a time- and

**Two-photon imaging shows transfer of a TfR1-VNAR/CD20
bispecific antibody to the brain parenchyma**

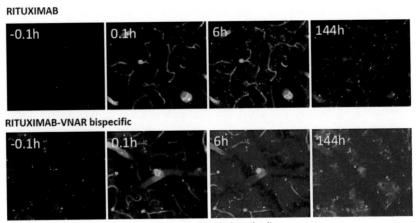

Time course after 4mg/kg, IV of Alexa488 labelled antibodies

FIGURE 3-1 Brain uptake of rituximab. Brain uptake of intravenous rituximab is greater, more rapid, and longer lasting when bound to the TfR1-VNAR Trojan horse (lower panel), compared to rituximab alone.
SOURCE: Presentation by Walsh, September 8, 2017.

dose-dependent manner and that it reduces amyloid levels in the cortex and hippocampus. CSF studies showed a similar reduction in amyloid beta (Aβ) levels, suggesting that CSF Aβ levels could be used as a surrogate marker of target engagement.

Chakravarthy and colleagues next repeated these studies in a rat model, which, because of its larger size, allowed them to conduct longitudinal structural and functional imaging studies. These studies showed a significant reduction in amyloid load, an increase in hippocampal volume, restoration of neuron connectivity, and no microhemorrhages. To assess how well the technology translated into larger animals, the researchers next moved to a dog model. Dogs naturally accumulate amyloid beta in their brains as they age and have measurable levels of CSF Aβ. After treatment with KAL-ABP-BBB, the dogs showed a pharmacokinetic profile, CSF to serum ratio, and decreases in CSF Aβ similar to the rat. The next step will be to test the compound in primates, said Chakravarthy.

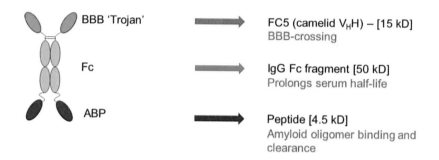

FIGURE 3-2 The fusion molecule KAL-ABP-BBB uses FC5 to initiate receptor-mediated transcytosis as a means of delivering the therapeutic peptide, ABP, to the brain.
SOURCE: Presentation by Chakravarthy, September 8, 2017.

Ruben Boado, cofounder of ArmaGen, described two Trojan horse therapeutics designed to treat mucopolysaccharidosis (MPS) types I and II, rare genetic diseases caused by deficiency of lysosomal enzymes that break down polysaccharide molecules called glycosaminoglycans (GAGs). Buildup of GAGs causes progressive multisystem dysfunction in children (Neufield and Muenzer, 2001). The most severe form of MPS I, known as Hurler syndrome, leads to profound neurocognitive decline (Shapiro et al., 2015). Patients with MPS II, also known as Hunter syndrome, may also develop neurological symptoms, including cognitive impairment (Whiteman and Kimura, 2017). Enzyme replacement therapy is the standard treatment. However, these enzymes do not cross the BBB, said Boado, so while they can be beneficial for relief of systemic symptoms they have little or no effect on CNS-related symptoms (Boado and Pardridge, 2017; Boado et al., 2013).

Boado said that for MPS I, ArmaGen generated a protein called AGT-181, which fused the missing enzyme, iduronidase (IDUA), with an antibody that targets the insulin receptor. The fusion protein has dual targeting effects for entry into the brain via the human insulin receptor and the mannose-6-phosphate receptor, which targets peripheral tissues (Boado et al., 2009, 2013). As shown in Figure 3-3, both IDUA and AGT-181 are taken up throughout peripheral tissue, but only the fusion protein enters the brain. Preliminary results from a phase II clinical study indicate that AGT-181 improves shoulder range of motion and reduces GAG buildup throughout the body, said Boado. In the CNS, AGT-181 improved or stabilized test scores across multiple cognitive domains and reduced

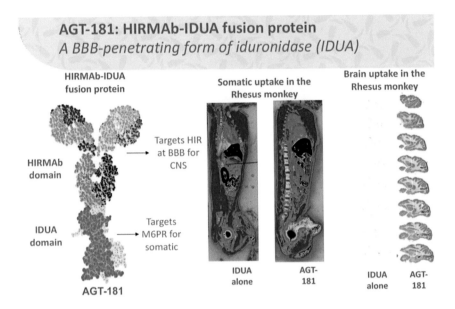

FIGURE 3-3 AGT-181 is generated by fusing iduronidase (IDUA) with an antibody to the human insulin receptor (HIR). The mannose-6-phosphate receptor (M6PR) enables distribution throughout peripheral tissues (central panel), and the HIR enables brain penetration (right panel). The right panel also shows that IDUA alone does not enter the brain, since it cannot cross the BBB.
SOURCES: Presentation by Boado, September 8, 2017. Reprinted with permission from Boado, R. J., and Pardridge, W. M. 2017. Brain and Organ Uptake in the Rhesus Monkey in Vivo of Recombinant Iduronidase Compared to an Insulin Receptor Antibody–Iduronidase Fusion Protein. *Molecular Pharmaceutics* 14(4):1271–1277. Copyright 2017 American Chemical Society.

brain atrophy, he said. He added that there is also evidence that the compound induces immune tolerance to IDUA, in contrast to treatment with enzyme replacement therapy, which can sometimes elicit a severe immune reaction. ArmaGen is also testing a similar compound for the treatment of MPS II, with similar results in early clinical trials, said Boado.

Cells and Exosomes: Harnessing Inflammatory Processes

A different approach to traversing the BBB uses immune cells, such as monocytes and macrophages, which are capable of infiltrating the brain in neuroinflammatory diseases such as Parkinson's disease (PD). Alexander Kabanov, Mescal Swaim Ferguson Distinguished Professor at the University of North Carolina at Chapel Hill, said that this technique was originally used to deliver antiretroviral therapy to the brain in a rodent model of human immunodeficiency virus (HIV)-associated brain disease (Dou et al., 2009). His lab took this approach further by using macrophages to deliver therapeutic "nanozymes" (small artificial enzymes) to inflammatory sites in the brains of PD mouse models (Zhao et al., 2011), reasoning that antioxidant enzymes would suppress the inflammatory response and protect neurons. Indeed, neuroinflammation was reduced, and neuroprotective responses increased, said Kabanov (Brynskikh et al., 2010).

Kabanov and colleagues have also shown that genetically modified macrophages can be used to transfer therapeutic genes into the brain (Haney et al., 2013). They transfected macrophages with the gene for glial cell derived neurotrophic factor and showed that these cells produced antiinflammatory, neuroprotective, and improved behavioral effects in a PD mouse model (Zhao et al., 2014). They went on to show that the enzymes were packaged into extracellular vesicles, called exosomes, secreted by the macrophages. These exosomes increase the persistence of the enzymes in the blood and facilitate the uptake of the nanozyme by neurons, said Kabanov (Haney et al., 2012). His lab has also shown that the uptake of exosomes is increased in the presence of brain inflammation, and that uptake is mediated, at least in part, by a protein on the exosome surface called lymphocyte function-associated antigen 1 (LFA-1), which binds to an intercellular adhesion molecule 1 (ICAM-1) on the surface of endothelial cells (Yuan et al., 2017). Kabanov suggested that understanding these mechanisms more fully may enable development of additional strategies to deliver to the brain therapeutic proteins, as well as DNA, small interfering RNA (siRNA), and messenger RNA (mRNA).

Viral Vectors

Viruses provide yet another versatile and powerful strategy to traverse the BBB and deliver proteins and genes to the brain, said Viviana Gradinaru. Adenoassociated viruses (AAVs) have been used in clinical trials to safely deliver therapeutic genes, via direct injection, to the brains of people with PD, which she said suggested the feasibility of this approach (Kaplitt et al., 2007). Gradinaru, however, said she wanted to use AAV as a vector to deliver multicolored gene labels to the brain as a way of mapping brain circuits, and she wanted to introduce these viral vectors systemically, which would require traversing the BBB. A paper published in 2009 showed that AAV9, when injected intravenously into neonatal mice, efficiently transduced neurons throughout the brain, although the efficiency was greatly reduced in adult mice (Foust et al., 2009). To overcome this roadblock, she and her team created libraries of AAV capsids (the outer coat of the viral particle) with different characteristics, and then selected those that made it through the BBB and efficiently transduced neurons and astrocytes in the brain (Deverman et al., 2016) (see Figure 3-4). Gradinaru said that by using different gene regulatory elements, it is also possible to target specific cells or regions of the brain for gene delivery (Chan et al., 2017).

An important unresolved question is whether gene therapy vectors will behave differently when confronted with a compromised BBB, such as in multiple sclerosis, inflammation, or brain tumors, said Gradinaru. She noted that a compromised BBB is not necessarily leakier because of fibrous tissue that could prevent the passage of small molecules. This will require more testing, she said.

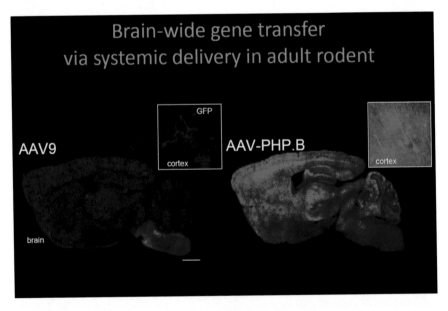

FIGURE 3-4 The novel genetically engineered adenoassociated virus, AAV-PHP.B, efficiently transduces neurons throughout the adult rodent brain, demonstrating its potential to deliver therapeutic molecules to the brain. For comparison, the left panel shows the low levels of in vivo gene transfer achieved when using the older, common AAV9 gene-vehicle.
SOURCE: Presentation by Gradinaru, September 8, 2017.

Focused Ultrasound

Focused ultrasound is yet another approach that has shown promise in disrupting the BBB to facilitate drug entry into the brain, said Alexandra Golby. As a neurosurgeon specializing in brain tumor surgery, Golby became interested in this technology because of the urgent need to improve treatments for brain tumors, which are difficult to resect owing to their infiltrative nature. And even though brain tumors may be associated with a disrupted BBB, they are less permeable to drugs, which limits efficacy, said Golby (Lockman et al., 2010).

While questions remain about the exact mechanisms by which focused ultrasound disrupts the BBB, Golby said the effects appear to be largely facilitated by microbubbles creating oscillations and vibrations that enhance the permeability of the brain-tumor barrier (Park et al., 2017). She noted that BBB disruption can occur in the absence of microbubbles; the microbubbles facilitate this and allow it to happen at lower power, thus minimizing damage.

The microbubbles may also carry a payload into the tumor, including chemotherapy agents, antibodies, nanoparticles, neuroprotective agents, and viruses, she added. The delivery of these agents has been advanced through the efforts of Nathan McDannold and others, who have fine tuned the magnitude of the BBB opening and the restoration of its closure, said Golby (Marty et al., 2012; Park et al., 2012). Indeed, she said it may be advantageous to close the BBB relatively quickly to protect the brain from toxins.

Golby described preclinical studies in a rat glioma model that showed that focused ultrasound increased both drug delivery and retention (Park et al., 2017) and improved survival (Aryal et al., 2013). Studies in macaque monkeys further showed that focused ultrasound can be targeted to open the BBB in a restricted area without causing tissue damage or functional impairment, she said (McDannold et al., 2012).

An Israeli company, Insightec, has received Food and Drug Administration (FDA) approval for a focused ultrasound device to do thermal ablations for movement disorders, said Golby. She added that the device can readily perform BBB opening as well. However, infrastructure requirements for the procedure are high: presently this procedure must be performed in an MRI scanner with a stereotactic head frame and a water bath for ultrasound transmission and cooling the scalp. Preoperative imaging is also needed to determine the exact bone thickness so the beams can be focused accurately. Golby suggested that for some indications, unfocused ultrasound may be useful, although this approach is less well developed.

BYPASSING THE BBB

While many mechanisms for traversing the BBB are under development, researchers seeking improved drug delivery to the CNS are also investigating methods that bypass the BBB altogether.

Intrathecal Injection

Intrathecal infusions can effectively deliver drugs to the subarachnoid space; however, since there is little penetration beyond the brain surface their use has been limited, according to Golby. Thorne said he has been trying to overcome problems with distribution of therapeutic molecules, such as antibodies. One approach Thorne has taken, in collaboration with Danica Stanimirovic, is to use single-domain antibodies, which are able to diffuse more readily in the brain. They have also tried CSF co-infusions of therapeutic molecules with substances such as mannitol that enhance distribution by increasing the access of some therapeutics to the perivascular spaces, leading to deeper brain penetration and more widespread distribution overall within the CNS.

Intranasal Delivery

Thorne has also explored using intranasal delivery to increase distribution of therapeutic antibodies throughout the CNS. He noted that many therapeutics (such as calcitonin for osteoporosis) are already approved and available that use intranasal administration to achieve systemic distribution since the nasal passages are highly vascularized. But his research has done much to expand further on how the intranasal route may be used to target the CNS specifically. He and others have shown in rodent models that intranasally delivered molecules are transported across the nasal epithelia to reach brain entry pathways associated with the olfactory and trigeminal nerves in the nasal mucosa, bypassing the BBB to achieve higher levels of macromolecules (e.g., labeled dextrans, antibodies, and antibody fragments) in perivascular spaces compared to intra-arterial administration (Lochhead et al., 2015). However, the olfactory mucosa in humans covers a much smaller area than in rodents, so further testing in primates and humans is necessary to determine the feasibility of this approach. Thorne and colleagues have tested intranasal administration of beta interferon—a drug approved for relapsing remitting multiple sclerosis—in cynomolgus monkeys and showed "fairly widespread distribution" with localization to appropriate brain regions (i.e., the basal ganglia); however, he acknowledged that this effect may not be completely generalizable so it will likely be necessary to examine on a case-by-case basis the distribution and CNS target concentrations of other drugs administered intranasally (Thorne et al., 2008). The intranasal route has also been used to administer exosomes, said Kabanov.

MODELING THE BBB

Development of novel biological and computational models of the BBB can contribute to facilitating translational research and understanding the dynamics of therapeutics once they are delivered to their nervous system target.

Spheroids as In Vitro Screening Tools

In vitro models of the BBB facilitate the discovery and development of new drugs to treat CNS diseases, said Choi-Fong Cho. Cho described a new platform for drug discovery using multicellular spheroids composed of all the important cells of the BBB: astrocytes in the core surrounded by pericytes and endothelial cells on the surface (Cho et al., 2017). She said these spheroids are extremely cost-effective and easily reproducible. Because they are created from human endothelial cells, they can provide extra support for moving a preclinical program into human clinical trials, she said. They are characterized by the expression of tight junctions and the function of efflux pumps, and certain receptors (such as the LRP-1 receptor) can mediate transcytosis of their ligands from the surface to the interior of the spheroid, enabling screening and prediction of molecules that can cross the BBB, she said. The platform is a high-throughput tool for studying molecular movement from the surface to the interior, enabling screening for molecules that can cross the BBB, Cho added.

Her lab has also used the model to test for BBB penetrating compounds. Compared to the commonly used transwell models of the BBB (Hatherell et al., 2011), the spheroid model is superior at reproducing and maintaining essential BBB properties and functions, said Cho. Her research showed a high level of angiopep-2 transport through their transwell insert over time, but the transwell insert also saw high penetration of the control (scrambled) peptide (Cho et al., 2017), highlighting the inherently leaky nature of the transwell system. The leakiness of the transwell system has been a long-standing problem with the model, and she said their findings are in line with previously published reports. Eric Schaeffer commented that other labs have reported good results using the transwell model and suggested that understanding the differences between these systems could provide valuable insight. Steven Hyman suggested that using human-induced pluripotent stem cells could avoid potential problems associated with immortalized cells.

Translational Pharmacokinetics Models

Mathematical models may also be useful to translate pharmacokinetics data from animal studies and predict how a compound will behave in humans, according to Dhaval Shah, assistant professor in the Department of Pharmaceutical Sciences at the State University of New York at Buffalo. His rationale for this approach is based on two beliefs: first, that molecules will behave similarly in humans and animals, and second, that the fundamental behavior of a system can be characterized mathematically. He suggested that the decision-making process for clinical translation would become more reliable by relying on mathematical models rather than one's hunch or gut feeling.

Shah and colleagues performed microdialysis experiments in rats, combined with sensitive enzyme-linked immunosorbent assay (ELISA) assays to understand and quantify the main determinants for protein therapeutics disposition, such as antibody-drug conjugates (Khot et al., 2017). They then used these data to develop a translational mathematical model. This model suggests, for example, that the brain–cerebrospinal fluid barrier may play an important role in transferring antibody molecules into the CSF, and that antibody concentrations vary among different compartments of the CSF circulatory system. Shah suggested that better understanding this process could help drug developers better understand how much drug is actually reaching targets in the brain and predict appropriate dosing.

4

Regulatory Considerations for Drugs That Traverse the Blood–Brain Barrier

Highlights

- Sponsors should seek regulatory advice early in clinical development (Manji, Whittaker).
- Areas of major concern to regulators include off-target effects, safety of long-term dosing, immunogenicity, and unintended consequences (Patel).
- Technologies that disrupt the blood–brain barrier raise other safety concerns regarding exposure of the brain to chemicals or toxins (Patel).
- Evaluating the safety profile of biologics can be particularly challenging as they may combine multiple components that will be delivered to the brain (Stanimirovic).
- Assessing the immunogenicity of biologics will usually require safety studies in at least one rodent and one nonrodent species (Schaeffer, Whittaker).
- Preclinical studies should focus not only on safety but also on efficacy (Bosetti).
- Since animal models may have limited reliability as tools for assessing human toxicity, multiple in vivo and in vitro studies may be required to establish a starting dose, followed by incremental dose increases (Chiocca, Whittaker).
- The acceptable safety threshold and the risk–benefit ratio for a therapeutic will vary depending on the condition being treated (Bosetti, Hunt).
- Focused ultrasound introduces many regulatory challenges because it combines a device, microbubbles, the therapeutic agent, and an imaging agent (Golby).

25

NOTE: These points were made by the individual speakers identified above; they are not intended to reflect a consensus among workshop participants.

Husseini Manji suggested that from a regulatory perspective, moving a therapy forward that involves novel methods for crossing the blood–brain barrier (BBB) enters into uncharted territory. Thus, he said, it makes sense to seek the advice of regulators early in the process. Matthew Whittaker concurred, adding that face-to-face meetings between sponsors and the clinical review team at the Food and Drug Administration (FDA) are critical to answer questions associated with trial design.

Vikram Patel, deputy director of the Division of Applied Regulatory Science in the Center for Drug Evaluation and Research at FDA, raised four areas of concern with the technologies discussed: off-target activity, safety of long-term dosing for chronic diseases, immunogenicity, and unintended consequences. For example, he noted that off-target activity could be particularly troublesome when using the transferrin or insulin receptors since they are ubiquitous. To ensure the safety of chronic dosing, more data will be needed. With regard to immunogenicity, he recalled that although checkpoint inhibitors appeared to be safe in preclinical models, when they were introduced in the clinic, patients died as a result of high-level immune activation that caused excessive, systemic autoimmune responses. He suggested that new technologies, such as humanized mouse models, may enable prediction of this reaction. There may also be other unexpected consequences to therapy with these novel therapeutics, he said.

Opening the BBB with focused ultrasound or other technologies raises other issues of particular relevance to regulators, said Patel. As mentioned earlier, for example, it may be desirable to close the BBB as soon as possible to limit exposure of the brain to chemicals or toxins other than the intended therapeutic compounds. Patel said that for some treatments, strategies may also be needed to keep drugs in the brain longer so that dosing can be less frequent, possibly resulting in a reduction of toxicity. Specific issues related to preclinical and clinical phases of development are discussed in more detail below.

PRECLINICAL ISSUES

Matthew Whittaker said that he and his colleagues at FDA evaluate the nonclinical data to determine if a study should proceed, and then inform clinical reviewers on the review team of potential risks that may exist. With biologics, unexpected challenges arise, said Douglas Hunt. The job of a company's regulatory affairs department is to try to project where things can go wrong, formulate questions that need answering to address specific challenges, and then look at the data to try to answer these questions and assess the risks and benefits, he said. Danica Stanimirovic noted that since Trojan horses are quite complex—usually at least bifunctional—and may combine antibodies, enzymes, and growth factors that will be delivered into the brain, evaluating safety may be particularly difficult.

Another potential complication that can affect both safety and efficacy of biologics is immunogenicity, said Eric Schaeffer. To avoid evoking strong immune reactions in preclinical models, different antibodies may be required for studies in rodents versus primates, he said. For example, human proteins may elicit a strong antibody response in rodents, which generally means that safety studies must be conducted in at least one rodent and one nonrodent species, said Whittaker. He said that sponsors address these kinds of issues in different ways with guidance from FDA. Patel noted that even with creative solutions and apparently adequate safety studies in animal models, there may still be surprises. Thus, sponsors must be prepared to carefully monitor safety in phase I studies, he said.

In addition to safety, Francesca Bosetti reminded workshop participants to also keep efficacy in mind. She said that preclinical, translational programs at the National Institute of Neurological Disorders and Stroke try to mimic as closely as possible the practices used in clinical trials, keeping in mind that outcome measures in clinical studies should reflect outcome measures that are used as end points in clinical trials. Hunt agreed, noting that in order to provide animal data on safety and efficacy relevant to humans, selecting the right model for preclinical studies requires not only that the therapeutic molecule crosses the BBB but also that it finds the correct receptor in the brain.

In terms of safety, the regulatory requirements for a drug intended for an orphan indication are no different than for any other drug, said Whittaker. Generally, this means that there must be an acceptable margin between the observed adverse effect level in animals versus the maximum dose that the sponsor intends to give humans, he said, noting that this includes adverse effects in the brain as well as in other organ systems throughout the body.

CLINICAL ISSUES

Moving from preclinical to clinical development, E. Antonio Chiocca, Harvey Cushing Professor of Neurosurgery at Harvard Medical School, expressed concern about using animal models for safety assessments, since animal models may have limited reliability as tools for assessing human toxicity. However, Whittaker commented that for first-in-human trials the only safety data available may have come from animal studies. One approach some sponsors have taken, he said, is to integrate all available in vivo and in vitro data to establish the minimal anticipated biological effect level, followed by incremental dose increases (Muller et al., 2009). Patel added that while a sign of toxicity in animal models may not be relevant to humans, it cannot be ignored and must be followed up with modeling and other studies.

Another concern about the use of animal models was raised by Bosetti, who noted that while small animals present fewer ethical challenges and are cheaper and widely available, they may lack relevance in terms of diffusion, since it is much easier to reach all areas of a smaller brain compared to a larger one. Bosetti added that the acceptable safety threshold for a therapeutic agent will vary depending on the condition being treated. For example, patients may accept a lower safety threshold for an aggressive lethal brain cancer than they would for a long-term neurological disease, she said. Thus, when evaluating a treatment such as focused ultrasound, she suggested that developers and regulators may need to consider the potential for long-term cognitive effects. Subtle cognitive effects would be difficult to detect in nonclinical studies, said Whittaker and Patel. Hunt suggested that a registry would likely be needed for long-term follow-up.

William Potter, senior advisor to the director at the National Institute of Mental Health, raised another safety issue that could come up in phase I clinical studies. For setting doses, it may be necessary to expose trial participants to radiolabeled tracers that indicate the concentrations of drug reaching relevant areas of the brain. To determine the risks of that exposure, Deepa Rao said that preclinical toxicology studies in animals would be the first step, and Patel added that in humans it would be important to use radioactive compounds with a relatively short half-life.

Once clearance is given by FDA to allow testing in humans, the risk–benefit ratio becomes the key point of discussion, said Patel. Hunt noted that the risk–benefit ratio is different for each indication. One challenge he cited in assessing risks and benefits for orphan indications is the appropriate clinical end point may be unclear. A bigger challenge in terms of conducting a clinical trial for an orphan indication is enrollment and how to deal with heterogeneity when the number of trial participants is small, he said.

Alexandra Golby said that she and her colleagues are in discussions with FDA to try to put together the first clinical trial of focused ultrasound with microbubbles to disrupt the BBB and deliver drugs. She added that this approach poses additional regulatory challenges since it combines a device, microbubbles, and an imaging agent, plus the drug that is being delivered. However, she noted that the devices (the device for thermal ablation and the microbubbles for imaging although neither has been approved for BBB opening) imaging agent, drugs, and microbubbles have already been approved for use. A regulatory package will also require substantial work to determine what volume of the brain can be safely targeted with this approach and whether repeated treatments can be delivered. And, most importantly, the right drugs are needed, she said. Therapeutic agents that have already been approved for other indications are being considered, Golby added.

While consideration of cost is not part of the FDA mandate, Hunt and others commented that costs are often of concern to people involved in drug development as well as to society as a whole. With the advent of more expensive technologies, he suggested that citizens will have to participate in decision making about which treatments should be subsidized. Patel suggested that one way to lower costs of clinical trials might be by developing and qualifying biomarkers.

5

Accelerating Research and Clinical Translation: Consortia and Public–Private Partnerships

Highlights

- Consortia and public–private partnerships (PPPs) can accelerate research by providing funding as well as by supporting collaboration across disciplines and stakeholder groups (Lisanby).

- The Innovative Medicines Initiative, a European Commission-industry partnership, funds two projects that may improve understanding of how to deliver therapeutics across the blood–brain barrier (BBB) (Stowasser).

- The BRAIN Initiative, a partnership of federal and nonfederal agencies in the United States that focuses on mapping brain circuits, funds research, and facilitates the development of PPPs relevant to the BBB (Talley).

- Wellcome supports research in the United Kingdom and internationally, but it has received few grant applications relevant to the BBB (Welchman).

- A newcomer in the biomedical research space, the Chan Zuckerberg Initiative, plans to fund research in neurodegeneration (Brose).

- Advancing innovative BBB research will require an increased focus on basic science, attracting more young researchers to the field, and supporting them to stay in the field (Brose, Gu, Lisanby, Talley, Thorne).

- Attracting the interest and expertise of investigators from outlying fields would encourage innovation in BBB science (Campany).

NOTE: These points were made by the individual speakers identified above; they are not intended to reflect a consensus among workshop participants.

Accelerating research on traversing the blood–brain barrier (BBB), and facilitating clinical translation of this promising science and these promising technologies, will require increasing collaboration across various stakeholder communities, including academia, industry, the private sector, and federal agencies, said Sarah Lisanby, director of the Division of Translational Research at the National Institute of Mental Health (NIMH). In a series of presentations, workshop participants representing an array of consortia and public–private partnerships (PPPs) established both by governmental and private agencies described how they have been instrumental in advancing research and development in other areas of neuroscience and suggested that their experiences could provide a roadmap for the BBB field.

CONSORTIA, FOUNDATIONS, AND PUBLIC–PRIVATE PARTNERSHIPS THAT SUPPORT ADVANCES IN SCIENTIFIC AND CLINICAL SCIENCE

Several collaborative efforts are under way to facilitate the development and clinical research of novel methods for delivery of therapeutics across the BBB. Ongoing projects in the United Stated and Europe provide lessons on what is needed to move the field forward and inform new funders who may provide novel approaches to catalyze research.

Innovative Medicines Initiative

The Innovative Medicines Initiative (IMI) is a European PPP of the European Commission and the European Federation of Pharmaceutical Industries and Associations (EFPIA).[1] Stowasser said that between 2008 and 2024, IMI anticipates investing €5 billion (nearly $6 billion) to accelerate drug development in Europe. Half of this investment is coming from the European Commission, with the other half from the pharmaceutical industry in the form of people and expertise. Academic partners are selected by a neutral panel through a highly competitive process, he said, and they

---

[1]See http://www.imi.europa.eu/about-imi/history-imi-story-so-far (accessed January 24, 2018).

work alongside industry partners in precompetitive space with a requirement that decisions are reached through consensus from all partners. Stowasser noted that another factor that enables IMI to move projects forward is clear, up-front understanding of how intellectual property is managed: each owner or developer of intellectual property maintains ownership (or joint ownership if multiple developers are involved).

Among about 60 ongoing IMI projects, Stowasser said two are relevant to the BBB. COMPACT (Collaboration on the Optimization of Macromolecular Pharmaceutical Access to Cellular Targets) aims to understand the intracellular uptake of biologics. This project has yielded new formulations for noninvasive delivery of macromolecules, a better understanding of the function of different barriers, and potential novel targets, said Stowasser. A second upcoming project on the BBB aims to discover and characterize new targets and transport mechanisms for brain delivery of therapeutics to treat neurodegenerative and metabolic diseases.

PPPs such as the IMI approach provide benefits for all stakeholders, said Stowasser. Academic researchers join and shape a vibrant, productive environment and gain development expertise while translating basic research into benefits for patients; pharmaceutical companies address bottlenecks in drug discovery by sharing and pooling data, knowledge, skills, and risks; and small and medium-sized enterprises build partnerships that enable them to perfect and advance their innovations. Lack of reproducibility, a common problem in academic research, is addressed by validating results at multiple research centers, said Stowasser.

The BRAIN Initiative

The Brain Research through Advancing Innovative Neurotechnologies (BRAIN) Initiative was launched in 2013 by President Barack Obama as a partnership of federal and nonfederal agencies and organizations focused on mapping all the circuits in the brain. Today the BRAIN Initiative includes foundations, independent research institutes, major research universities, and industry partners, and it has been supported by more than $150 million for research.[2]

Edmund Talley said that the BRAIN Initiative interfaces with strategies for crossing the BBB because of their relevance to issues of accessing and understanding circuit activity and modulating circuits. For example, he noted that the neurovascular unit is a critical component that regulates

---

[2]See https://www.braininitiative.nih.gov (accessed January 24, 2018).

circuit activity (Ivanova et al., 2016). Talley said that the BRAIN Initiative exemplifies how the National Institutes of Health (NIH) can play an important role in establishing PPPs because of its access to the research community and understanding of where research is moving in the future. Moreover, NIH serves as a neutral third party, able to convene and liaise among academics and industry scientists. This has been particularly important in advancing research in the area of neuromodulation, he said, which, like the technologies discussed for traversing the BBB, requires the collaboration of multiple stakeholders from the pharmaceutical and device industries and thus has a complicated intellectual property and regulatory landscape. For example, the National Institute of Neurological Disorders and Stroke (NINDS) was interested in repurposing existing devices for new indications, and was able to convince companies that it was in their interest to share preexisting safety data on their devices with investigators funded by the BRAIN Initiative, and to put information about their devices on the BRAIN Initiative website. They also set up a template research agreement for companies to use as a starting point for negotiations over intellectual property, said Talley.

Wellcome

Private funders have also played important roles in supporting research. For example, Wellcome,[3] which has an endowment of about $30 billion, invests approximately $1.2 billion per year to advance the development of technologies for treatment and diagnostics to improve human health, said Andrew Welchman, head of neuroscience and mental health at the trust. Their grant-funding portfolio includes about £500 million (about $650 million) for neuroscience and mental health. Only a small fraction of that has supported research on the BBB; however, Welchman suggested that there is an opportunity to increase funding in that space. He noted that there have been few grant applications pertaining to the BBB. In addition to providing individual fellowships and investigator awards, Wellcome supports interdisciplinary teams working at the interface of science, technology, and innovation, he said.

Wellcome funds internationally and works in partnership with other funders, both governmental and nongovernmental, said Welchman. It re-

---

[3]See https://wellcome.ac.uk (accessed January 24, 2018).

cently hosted a workshop on academic–industry partnerships, which focused on overcoming barriers to innovation, derisking investments, and leveraging the expertise in academia and industry.

Chan Zuckerberg Initiative

One of the newest philanthropic initiatives in the biomedical research space is the Chan Zuckerberg Initiative (CZI).[4] Science is one of CZI's three major areas of interest, along with education and policy, said Katja Brose, science program officer at CZI. Its efforts will be focused on basic biomedical science where more financial support, advocacy, and platform development are needed to break the bottlenecks that have slowed progress, she said.

A feature that sets CZI apart from other funders is its world-class technology engineering team. By assembling top engineers from areas outside of the scientific community who have experience managing and interpreting enormous quantities of disparate data, CZI hopes to leverage its expertise in partnership with scientists to advance the development of enabling tools and technologies that can drive innovation in biomedicine, said Brose. It has identified neurodegeneration and biological imaging and computation as two areas of particular interest. In the area of neurodegeneration, for example, it plans to bring together engineers, computer scientists, and cell biologists to explore mechanisms of neurodegeneration in novel ways, said Brose. One of its other early-stage efforts has been to join the Human Cell Atlas (HCA) Project consortium, which aims to use new technologies around single-cell sequencing, next-gene sequencing, imaging, and other technologies to develop a foundational atlas of every cell in the human body. CZI provides funding for several aspects of the project. It is collaborating with scientists and engineers at other research institutions to build a data coordination platform, and it is working with HCA scientists to develop new tools and technologies for the entire scientific community, said Brose.

Brose said that CZI is also committed to supporting the next generation of scientists by changing the culture and institutional context around rewards and incentives in academia, which will give young scientists the freedom to be innovative and open minded.

---

[4]See https://chanzuckerberg.com (accessed January 24, 2018).

XPRIZE Foundation

Grant Campany, a senior director at the XPRIZE Foundation,[5] offered an alternative approach to problem solving, what the XPRIZE Foundation calls incentivized competition. The XPRIZE Foundation issues a challenge, defining very explicitly what it is looking for in terms of a solution, said Campany. It assembles an international team of key opinion leaders in the scientific community with specific types of expertise to evaluate submissions and the teams submitting them. The teams progress through several rounds of judging, with clear milestones that must be reached along the way, culminating in a large cash prize. For example, Campany recently ran a prize competition to develop a portable, wireless technology to monitor and diagnose health conditions and thus expand access to health care and better use limited health care resources. He said 300 teams from leading research institutions around the world vied for the prize, and after 4 years and extensive testing of prototypes, two teams were selected as winners, taking home several million dollars.

Campany said the prize approach helped accelerate the path to getting these devices commercialized. The advantages of this approach, he said, are that competitors are not restricted by current ways of approaching a problem, and doors are opened to collaboration. He added, however, that to be qualified as an XPRIZE, the end point must be well articulated, which can be challenging for basic science questions.

Kelsie Timbie of the Focused Ultrasound Foundation suggested a related funding model (without the aspect of a prize)[6] that combines competition with collaboration by selecting a disease model and metrics and then inviting participants to test their particular therapeutic agent or treatment. She said that this approach accommodates different delivery mechanisms and multiple disease models for the same disease, and this approach has made it easier to decide how to move forward, particularly with early-stage research.

APPLYING THE CONSORTIA MODEL TO BBB RESEARCH

Following the session on consortia and PPPs, Sarah Lisanby asked if a consortium were to be established for the BBB, who its members would

---

[5]See https://www.xprize.org (accessed January 24, 2018).
[6]See https://www.fusfoundation.org (accessed January 24, 2018).

be, what they would contribute, and what they would gain. Berislav Zlokovic advocated including people from multiple fields, such as vascular biologists, geneticists, scientists who focus on tau and amyloid beta, and clinical specialists.

Balancing Basic Science, Translational, and Clinical Research

Eric Schaeffer commented that the membership of a consortium would differ depending on the goal. For example, building basic science programs would require a longer timeline and different scientists, in comparison to a consortium aiming to move as rapidly as possible into therapeutic applications. Both are needed, he said. However, Danica Stanimirovic suggested that it may be a fallacy to divide basic science, applied science, and drug delivery into silos rather than thinking of them along a continuum. Consortia need to develop funding mechanisms that have a long-term perspective and enable development through that continuum, she said.

Consortia and other funders represented at the workshop ranged from those that are particularly adept at supporting foundational research, such the BRAIN Initiative and Wellcome, to those focusing on clinical outcomes, such as IMI. Welchman noted that while most of what Wellcome funds is in the basic sciences, there is also value in pursuing applications of those discoveries for the treatment of human diseases.

For riskier scientific endeavors, increased funding and education are needed, said Brose. But more importantly, the quality of the work must improve. For this, organizations such as CZI and XPRIZE may play a complementary role, funding projects submitted by individuals and groups that may be less likely to apply to more traditional funding organizations, said Lisanby. She noted that investing in basic science is an important part of the NIMH mission; Talley said the same is true at NINDS. In fact, he said that applications in basic neurobiology have a better chance of being funded, and at a higher pay line, than those submitted with a focus on a specific disease. Talley added that the potential for basic neuroscience is unprecedented. The ability to study single cells and to look at the diversity across the vasculature in the context of different disease states, as well as the potential for developing new models, have fueled tremendous excitement in the field, he said.

Chenghua Gu of Harvard Medical School, among others, advocated for an increased focus on basic science to expand the number of mechanisms that could be targeted. Stowasser said that in his opinion, the key is to recognize the problem, bring together the right people, and be ambitious. Welchman agreed, adding that having good baselines across different experiments will encourage the emergence of innovation.

Training and Attracting Scientists to BBB Research

Thorne suggested that funders establish centers of excellence in BBB science, with programs that would support the training of BBB scientists and provide incentives for them to stay in the field. For example, he suggested a three-tiered system that could provide funding for graduate studies, after which successful trainees would have priority for postdoctoral fellowships. Those who stay in the BBB field for their postdoctoral fellowship could then compete preferentially for seed financing to set up a new lab. This would expand the field by producing a cohort of BBB scientists, and the effort could also build up critical infrastructure, he said. Brose, however, suggested that establishing a program on BBB science may be too narrow, shutting out scientists who could bring needed expertise, ideas, and tools to the field. She suggested that such a program could be built around the topic of neurodegeneration, with BBB a component of that.

To attract more young scientists to the field, Gu advocated increased visibility for the novel, exciting work being done in the field. Steven Hyman noted that glia and endothelial cells were not considered interesting until research by Ben Barres, professor of neurobiology at Stanford, showed that they were important players in neurodegenerative disease.

Robert Thorne agreed that researchers in this field occupy a unique interface. Even though there is an International Brain Barrier Society and a number of thriving research conferences, there are probably fewer than 2,000 scientists in the field, he said. Moreover, BBB research has been conducted in silos, added Brose. She argued for engaging other disciplines, such as cell biology and engineering, into the research enterprise. Thorne agreed that while the field is small, it is truly multidisciplinary, comprising physicists, modelers, immunologists, cell biologists, and neuroscientists, while straddling basic and applied science.

The nature of this multidisciplinary science surrounding the central nervous system (CNS) barriers field has probably posed a problem in identifying just which departments or schools would make the best home for highly qualified CNS barriers scientists. He also suggested that the diffuse nature of the field can make it less appealing for federal funding agencies because there are often not well-defined study sections with the right fit and expertise to review grants that focus on CNS barriers work. Lisanby noted that small fields can benefit from cooperation and forming of consortia across groups.

Campany added another element to the equation: the importance of focusing attention on a problem and creating interest from a pool of talented individuals in outlying fields. Competition can encourage this, he said, bringing new insights and new ways of thinking into a problem. Not everyone agreed on the value of competitive models. William Potter suggested that competition gets in the way of progress and wastes resources. He supported international cooperative efforts as an alternative. Andrew Welchman elaborated on international collaborative awards, noting that teams funded by Wellcome bring together purely academic teams or teams of both academic and industry scientists. To secure funding from Wellcome, the principal investigator would have to be located in the United Kingdom, Ireland, or a lower- or middle-income country, he said. Coapplicants, however, can be located anywhere.

Additional Focus on Delivery and Regulatory Science

Thorne suggested that a roadblock to the treatment of brain disorders has been the pharmaceutical industry's lack of appreciation for delivery science as opposed to drug development. Investments through consortia and PPPs could remedy this, he said. Regulatory science represents another research area that is underappreciated by the academic community, said Talley. The field could benefit from increased research in this area, he said, noting that NIH and NINDS would welcome investigator-initiated proposals in this area. He also noted that the BRAIN Initiative plans to fund studies to better understand the biophysics underlying invasive devices, which will have substantial regulatory implications. The IMI also holds a regulatory forum every year to identify topics that need to be addressed in regulatory science.

FINAL THOUGHTS

The purpose of this workshop, according to Steven Hyman, was to bring together industry, government, foundations, patient groups, and academics to discuss important issues, gaps, and bottlenecks in the neurosciences, especially those related to the BBB, and to share ideas for possible solutions to outstanding questions. Indeed, the workshop discussions identified many unanswered questions.

William Potter suggested that advancing understanding of the BBB could be achieved through a systematic evaluation and prioritization of tools. For example, he suggested that the technology already exists with positron emission topography imaging and radiolabeled ligands to quantify a biologic agent as it enters the brain, yet these tools are not being used for this purpose. As a result, even after investments of billions of dollars, studies conclude with no interpretable data about dosing, he said.

Welchman compared the problems discussed at the workshop to the moon shot. The technology involved in going to the moon required bringing many elements together. Here, many tools have been discussed; now the challenge is to integrate them, he said.

A

References

Aryal, M., N. Vykhodtseva, Y. Z. Zhang, J. Park, and N. McDannold. 2013. Multiple treatments with liposomal doxorubicin and ultrasound–induced disruption of blood–tumor and blood–brain barriers improve outcomes in a rat glioma model. *Journal of Controlled Release* 169(1–2):103–111.

Boado, R. J., and W. M. Pardridge. 2017. Brain and organ uptake in the rhesus monkey in vivo of recombinant iduronidase compared to an insulin receptor antibody-iduronidase fusion protein. *Molecular Pharmaceutics* 14(4):1271–1277.

Boado, R. J., E. K. Hui, J. Z. Lu, and W. M. Pardridge. 2009. Agt–181: Expression in cho cells and pharmacokinetics, safety, and plasma iduronidase enzyme activity in rhesus monkeys. *Journal of Biotechnology* 144(2):135–141.

Boado, R. J., E. K. Hui, J. Z. Lu, R. K. Sumbria, and W. M. Pardridge. 2013. Blood–brain barrier molecular Trojan horse enables imaging of brain uptake of radioiodinated recombinant protein in the rhesus monkey. *Bioconjugate Chemistry* 24(10):1741–1749.

Brynskikh, A. M., Y. Zhao, R. L. Mosley, S. Li, M. D. Boska, N. L. Klyachko, A. V. Kabanov, H. E. Gendelman, and E. V. Batrakova. 2010. Macrophage delivery of therapeutic nanozymes in a murine model of Parkinson's disease. *Nanomedicine* 5(3):379–396.

Chan, G. N., R. A. Evans, D. B. Banks, E. V. Mesev, D. S. Miller, and R. E. Cannon. 2017. Selective induction of P-glycoprotein at the CNS barriers during symptomatic stage of an ALS animal model. *Neuroscience Letters* 639:103–113.

Cho, C. F., J. M. Wolfe, C. M. Fadzen, D. Calligaris, K. Hornburg, E. A. Chiocca, N. Y. R. Agar, B. L. Pentelute, and S. E. Lawler. 2017. Blood–brain barrier spheroids as an in vitro screening platform for brain-penetrating agents. *Nature Communications* 8:15623.

Deane, R., S. Du Yan, R. K. Submamaryan, B. LaRue, S. Jovanovic, E. Hogg, D. Welch, L. Manness, C. Lin, J. Yu, H. Zhu, J. Ghiso, B. Frangione, A. Stern, A. M. Schmidt, D. L. Armstrong, B. Arnold, B. Liliensiek, P. Nawroth, F.

Hofman, M. Kindy, D. Stern, and B. Zlokovic. 2003. RAGE mediates amyloid-beta peptide transport across the blood–brain barrier and accumulation in brain. *Nature Medicine* 9(7):907–913.

Deverman, B. E., P. L. Pravdo, B. P. Simpson, S. R. Kumar, K. Y. Chan, A. Banerjee, W. L. Wu, B. Yang, N. Huber, S. P. Pasca, and V. Gradinaru. 2016. CRE-dependent selection yields AAV variants for widespread gene transfer to the adult brain. *Nature Biotechnology* 34(2):204–209.

Dou, H., C. B. Grotepas, J. M. McMillan, C. J. Destache, M. Chaubal, J. Werling, J. Kipp, B. Rabinow, and H. E. Gendelman. 2009. Macrophage delivery of nanoformulated antiretroviral drug to the brain in a murine model of neuroaids. *Journal of Immunology* 183(1):661–669.

Foust, K. D., E. Nurre, C. L. Montgomery, A. Hernandez, C. M. Chan, and B. K. Kaspar. 2009. Intravascular AAV9 preferentially targets neonatal neurons and adult astrocytes. *Nature Biotechnology* 27(1):59–65.

Griffin, J. H., B. V. Zlokovic, and L. O. Mosnier. 2015. Activated protein C: Biased for translation. *Blood* 125(19):2898–2907.

Griffin, J. H., J. A. Fernandez, P. D. Lyden, and B. V. Zlokovic. 2016. Activated protein C promotes neuroprotection: Mechanisms and translation to the clinic. *Thrombosis Research* 141(Suppl 2):S62–S64.

Haney, M. J., P. Suresh, Y. Zhao, G. D. Kanmogne, I. Kadiu, M. Sokolsky–Papkov, N. L. Klyachko, R. L. Mosley, A. V. Kabanov, H. E. Gendelman, and E. V. Batrakova. 2012. Blood–borne macrophage–neural cell interactions hitchhike on endosome networks for cell–based nanozyme brain delivery. *Nanomedicine* 7(6):815–833.

Haney, M. J., Y. Zhao, E. B. Harrison, V. Mahajan, S. Ahmed, Z. He, P. Suresh, S. D. Hingtgen, N. L. Klyachko, R. L. Mosley, H. E. Gendelman, A. V. Kabanov, and E. V. Batrakova. 2013. Specific transfection of inflamed brain by macrophages: A new therapeutic strategy for neurodegenerative diseases. *PLoS ONE* 8(4):e61852.

Hatherell, K., P. O. Couraud, I. A. Romero, B. Weksler, and G. J. Pilkington. 2011. Development of a three-dimensional, all-human in vitro model of the blood–brain barrier using mono-, co-, and tri-cultivation transwell models. *Journal of Neuroscience Methods* 199(2):223–229.

Ivanova, E., C. W. Yee, and B. T. Sagdullaev. 2016. Leveraging optogenetic-based neurovascular circuit characterization for repair. *Neurotherapeutics* 13(2):341–347.

Jones, A. R., and E. V. Shusta. 2007. Blood–brain barrier transport of therapeutics via receptor-mediation. *Pharmaceutical Research* 24(9):1759–1771.

Kaplitt, M. G., A. Feigin, C. Tang, H. L. Fitzsimons, P. Mattis, P. A. Lawlor, R. J. Bland, D. Young, K. Strybing, D. Eidelberg, and M. J. During. 2007. Safety and tolerability of gene therapy with an adeno-associated virus (AAV) borne GAD gene for Parkinson's disease: An open label, phase I trial. *Lancet* 369(9579):2097–2105.

Khot, A., J. Tibbitts, D. Rock, and D. K. Shah. 2017. Development of a translational physiologically based pharmacokinetic model for antibody-drug conjugates: A case study with T-DM1. *AAPS Journal* 19(6):1715–1734.

Lochhead, J. J., D. J. Wolak, M. E. Pizzo, and R. G. Thorne. 2015. Rapid transport within cerebral perivascular spaces underlies widespread tracer distribution in the brain after intranasal administration. *Journal of Cerebral Blood Flow & Metabolism* 35(3):371–381.

Lockman, P. R., R. K. Mittapalli, K. S. Taskar, V. Rudraraju, B. Gril, K. A. Bohn, C. E. Adkins, A. Roberts, H. R. Thorsheim, J. A. Gaasch, S. Huang, D. Palmieri, P. S. Steeg, and Q. R. Smith. 2010. Heterogeneous blood-tumor barrier permeability determines drug efficacy in experimental brain metastases of breast cancer. *Clincal Cancer Research* 16(23):5664–5678.

Marty, B., B. Larrat, M. Van Landeghem, C. Robic, P. Robert, M. Port, D. Le Bihan, M. Pernot, M. Tanter, F. Lethimonnier, and S. Meriaux. 2012. Dynamic study of blood–brain barrier closure after its disruption using ultrasound: A quantitative analysis. *Journal of Cerebral Blood Flow & Metabolism* 32(10):1948–1958.

McDannold, N., C. D. Arvanitis, N. Vykhodtseva, and M. S. Livingstone. 2012. Temporary disruption of the blood–brain barrier by use of ultrasound and microbubbles: Safety and efficacy evaluation in rhesus macaques. *Cancer Research* 72(14):3652–3663.

Muller, P. Y., M. Milton, P. Lloyd, J. Sims, and F. R. Brennan. 2009. The minimum anticipated biological effect level (MABEL) for selection of first human dose in clinical trials with monoclonal antibodies. *Current Opinion in Biotechnology* 20(6):722–729.

Neufield, E., and J. Muenzer. 2001. The mucopolysaccharidoses. In *The metabolic and molecular bases of inherited disease*, edited by C. Scriver, A. Beaudet, D. Valle, and W. Sly. New York: McGraw–Hill Companies. Pp. 3421–3452.

Pardridge, W. M. 2006. Molecular Trojan horses for blood–brain barrier drug delivery. *Current Opinion in Pharmacology* 6(5):494–500.

Park, J., Y. Zhang, N. Vykhodtseva, F. A. Jolesz, and N. J. McDannold. 2012. The kinetics of blood–brain barrier permeability and targeted doxorubicin delivery into brain induced by focused ultrasound. *Journal of Controlled Release* 162(1):134–142.

Park, J., M. Aryal, N. Vykhodtseva, Y. Z. Zhang, and N. McDannold. 2017. Evaluation of permeability, doxorubicin delivery, and drug retention in a rat brain tumor model after ultrasound-induced blood–tumor barrier disruption. *Journal of Controlled Release* 250:77–85.

Shapiro, E. G., I. Nestrasil, K. Rudser, K. Delaney, V. Kovac, A. Ahmed, B. Yund, P. J. Orchard, J. Eisengart, G. R. Niklason, J. Raiman, E. Mamak, M. J. Cowan, M. Bailey–Olson, P. Harmatz, S. P. Shankar, S. Cagle, N. Ali, R. D. Steiner, J. Wozniak, K. O. Lim, and C. B. Whitley. 2015. Neurocognition across the spectrum of mucopolysaccharidosis type I: Age, severity, and treatment. *Molecular Genetics and Metabolism* 116(1–2):61–68.

Thorne, R. G., L. R. Hanson, T. M. Ross, D. Tung, and W. H. Frey, 2nd. 2008. Delivery of interferon–beta to the monkey nervous system following intranasal administration. *Neuroscience* 152(3):785–797.

Whiteman, D. A., and A. Kimura. 2017. Development of idursulfase therapy for mucopolysaccharidosis type II (Hunter syndrome): The past, the present and the future. *Drug Design, Development and Therapy* 11:2467–2480.

Winkler, E. A., Y. Nishida, A. P. Sagare, S. V. Rege, R. D. Bell, D. Perlmutter, J. D. Sengillo, S. Hillman, P. Kong, A. R. Nelson, J. S. Sullivan, Z. Zhao, H. J. Meiselman, R. B. Wendy, J. Soto, E. D. Abel, J. Makshanoff, E. Zuniga, D. C. De Vivo, and B. V. Zlokovic. 2015. GLUT1 reductions exacerbate Alzheimer's disease vasculo–neuronal dysfunction and degeneration. *Nature Neuroscience* 18(4):521–530.

Yuan, D., Y. Zhao, W. A. Banks, K. M. Bullock, M. Haney, E. Batrakova, and A. V. Kabanov. 2017. Macrophage exosomes as natural nanocarriers for protein delivery to inflamed brain. *Biomaterials* 142:1–12.

Zhao, Y., M. J. Haney, N. L. Klyachko, S. Li, S. L. Booth, S. M. Higginbotham, J. Jones, M. C. Zimmerman, R. L. Mosley, A. V. Kabanov, H. E. Gendelman, and E. V. Batrakova. 2011. Polyelectrolyte complex optimization for macrophage delivery of redox enzyme nanoparticles. *Nanomedicine* 6(1):25–42.

Zhao, Y., M. J. Haney, R. Gupta, J. P. Bohnsack, Z. He, A. V. Kabanov, and E. V. Batrakova. 2014. GDNF–transfected macrophages produce potent neuroprotective effects in Parkinson's disease mouse model. *PLoS ONE* 9(9):e106867.

Zhao, Z., A. R. Nelson, C. Betsholtz, and B. V. Zlokovic. 2015. Establishment and dysfunction of the blood–brain barrier. *Cell* 163(5):1064–1078.

Zlokovic, B. V. 2011. Neurovascular pathways to neurodegeneration in Alzheimer's disease and other disorders. *Nature Review Neuroscience* 12(12):723–738.

B

Workshop Agenda

**Enabling Novel Treatments for Nervous System Disorders
by Improving Methods for Traversing the Blood–Brain Barrier:
A Workshop**

September 8, 2017
Keck Center of the National Academies
500 Fifth Street, NW | Washington, DC

Background:

The blood–brain barrier (BBB) presents a special challenge to the development of therapeutics for many central nervous system (CNS) disorders. Far from acting simply as a physical barrier, the BBB is a complex dynamic system involving several cell types, passive and active transport mechanisms, and adaptive function to control the exchange of substances between the blood and the CNS. Few therapeutic agents readily traverse the BBB to reach the brain or spinal cord, including most small-molecule drugs and the vast majority of large molecules, such as proteins. Several research groups are exploiting intrinsic BBB transport mechanisms, such as molecular Trojan horses, and exploring technologies, such as chemical modifications and physical disruption, to test delivery of therapeutic agents to the CNS. Such strategies may greatly increase the armamentarium of potential drugs for treating psychiatric and neurological disorders. This public workshop will bring together key experts from academia, government, the biotechnology and pharmaceutical sector, disease-focused organizations, and other interested stakeholders to explore current development of novel methods for traversing the

BBB to deliver therapeutics for nervous system disorders and to identify potential opportunities for moving the field forward.

Workshop Objectives:

- Provide an overview of current knowledge on the role of the BBB biology and delivery mechanisms examining gaps in our current knowledge that future research may address.
- Discuss BBB passive and active mechanisms that challenge development and delivery of effective therapeutic interventions to CNS targets.
- Highlight current data and innovative approaches for delivery of therapeutics across the BBB harnessing methods, including chemical modifications, Trojan horse approaches, physical targeting and disruption, nanoparticles, ultrasound, and other technologies.
- Explore potential opportunities for catalyzing development of novel treatments that cross the BBB—from the preclinical to the clinical phase—with an emphasis on risks, levers, and potential collaborative efforts among sectors.

September 8, 2017, Room 100

8:00 a.m.   **Welcome and Overview of Workshop**
                 HUSSEINI MANJI, Janssen Research &
                 Development, LLC (Co-Chair)
                 DANICA STANIMIROVIC, National Research
                 Council of Canada (Co-Chair)

OPENING TALKS

Session Objectives:

- Provide background information about BBB biology, including its function in health and disease states and active and passive mechanisms challenging delivery of therapeutics to the CNS.
- Review different mechanisms and modes for traversing the BBB for the purpose of therapeutic delivery to the CNS.
- Highlight gaps in our understanding of BBB biology and transport mechanisms for delivery of therapeutics to the brain.

8:10 a.m.   **Introduction**
HUSSEINI MANJI, Janssen Research &
Development, LLC (Moderator)

8:20 a.m.   **BBB Structure, Function, and Pathology**
BERISLAV ZLOKOVIC, University of Southern
California

8:35 a.m.   **Modes of Traversing and Overcoming the BBB**
WILLIAM PARDRIDGE, University of California,
Los Angeles

8:50 a.m.   **Discussion**

9:05 a.m.   ***Break***

SESSION 1: TRAVERSING THE BBB: MODALITIES AND TECHNOLOGIES FOR BRAIN DELIVERY

Session Objectives:

- Describe current understanding of modalities for traversing the BBB.
- Survey innovative technologies—including Trojan horse approaches, physical targeting and disruption, nanoparticles, and ultrasound—for delivery of therapeutics to the CNS.
- Discuss desirable characteristics for development of new technologies for traversing the BBB.

9:20 a.m.   **Session Overview**
ERIC SCHAEFFER, Janssen Research &
Development, LLC (Moderator)

9:30 a.m.   **Presentations**
FRANK WALSH, Ossianix
VIVIANA GRADINARU, California Institute of
Technology

ROBERT THORNE, University of Wisconsin–
    Madison
ALEXANDER KABANOV, University of North
    Carolina at Chapel Hill
CHOI-FONG CHO, Brigham and Women's
    Hospital

10:30 a.m.   **Discussion**

11:00 a.m.   ***Break***

SESSION 2: TRAVERSING THE BBB: PRECLINICAL TO CLINICAL TRANSLATION

Session Objectives:

- Discuss the translation—from late preclinical work to clinical trials—of delivery strategies for traversing the BBB, including delivery of synthetic molecules, biologics, and gene therapy.
- Describe the limitations of current methods for traversing the BBB and identify research and other potential next steps that would move the field forward.

11:15 a.m.   **Session Overview**
    DANICA STANIMIROVIC, National Research
        Council of Canada (Co-Moderator)
    E. ANTONIO CHIOCCA, Harvard Medical School
        (Co-Moderator)

11:25 a.m.   **Presentations**
    BALU CHAKRAVARTHY, National Research
        Council of Canada
    ALEXANDRA GOLBY, Brigham and Women's
        Hospital
    RUBEN BOADO, ArmaGen
    DAHAVALKUMAR SHAH, State University of
        New York at Buffalo

12:25 p.m.   **Discussion**

12:55 p.m.   ***Lunch***

PANEL 1: REGULATORY CONSIDERATIONS IN DEVELOPMENT OF METHODS FOR TRAVERSING THE BBB

Session Objectives:

- Discuss approaches, tools, and lessons learned from other regulatory domains that may advance the development and translation of novel methods to traverse the BBB.
- Identify specific barriers and opportunities in the regulatory domain related to the development and application of methods for traversing the BBB.
- Explore issues related to critical attributes and potency assays; safety, including immunogenicity and CNS toxicity; and animal models, including appropriate species selection.
- Explore best practices and strategies to facilitate regulatory consideration of novel technologies for traversing the BBB.

1:40 p.m. **Session Overview**
FRANCESCA BOSETTI, National Institute of Neurological Disorders and Stroke (Moderator)

1:50 p.m. **Panel Remarks**
DOUGLAS HUNT, ArmaGen
VIKRAM PATEL, Food and Drug Administration

2:20 p.m. **Discussion**

2:40 p.m. ***Break***

PANEL 2: ACCELERATING RESEARCH AND CLINICAL TRANSLATION—CONSORTIA AND PUBLIC–PRIVATE PARTNERSHIPS

Session Objectives:

- Identify specific barriers and opportunities for increased coordinating among ongoing efforts in academia, the private sector, and federal agencies.
- Brainstorm potential collaborative projects that could be submitted through current or planned mechanisms.
- Explore novel mechanisms for catalyzing innovative technologies for traversing the BBB through new public–private partnerships and consortia, including discussion of potential practical next steps.

2:55 p.m.   **Session Overview**
             SARAH H. LISANBY, National Institute of Mental
             Health (MODERATOR)

3:05 p.m.   **Reflecting on the Workshop: Challenges and
             Emerging Opportunities for Development of
             Innovative Methods to Traverse the BBB**
             ERIC SCHAEFFER, Session 1 Moderator
             E. ANTONIO CHIOCCA, Session 2 Co-Moderator
             FRANCESCA BOSETTI, Panel 1 Moderator

3:30 p.m.   **Panel Remarks**
             BERND STOWASSER, Sanofi
             ANDREW WELCHMAN, Wellcome Trust
             EDMUND TALLEY, National Institute for
                 Neurological Disorders and Stroke/BRAIN
                 Initiative
             KATJA BROSE, Chan Zuckerberg Initiative
             GRANT CAMPANY, XPRIZE Foundation

5:00 p.m.   **Discussion**

5:30 p.m.   ***Adjourn Workshop***

C

Registered Attendees

Neeraj Agarwal
National Eye Institute

Diaa Ahmed
Helway University

Mark Allegretta
National Multiple Sclerosis
Society

Susan Amara
National Institute of Mental
Health

Forest Andrews
Eli Lilly and Company

Shelli Avenevoli
National Institute of Mental
Health

Frank Avenilla
National Institute of Mental
Health

David Banach
AbbVie, Inc.

Abdulai Barrie
Department of Chemical and
Biological Sciences,
Montgomery College,
Germantown, Maryland

Isle Bastille
Harvard Medical School

William Beckett
William Beckett & Associates

Virginia Berry
Amgen

Julia Berzhanskaya
National Institutes of Health

Ruben Boado
ArmaGen

Karen Boisvert
AbbVie Inc.

Lizbet Boroughs
Association of American
Universities

Francesca Bosetti
National Institute of
   Neurological Disorders and
   Stroke

Katja Brose
Chan Zuckerberg Initiative

Michael T. Brown
GE Global Research

Gregory Busse
Takeda Pharmaceuticals

Grant Campany
XPRIZE Foundation

Rosa Canet-Aviles
Foundation for the National
   Institutes of Health

Mark Carol
Sonacare Medical

Randall Carter
GE Global Research

Martin Case
Janssen Research &
   Development, LLC

Balu Chakravarthy
National Research Council of
   Canada

Ying Chan
AbbVie Inc.

Ellen Chi
Janssen Research &
   Development, LLC

Sylvia Chin-Caplan
Law Office of Sylvia Chin-
   Caplan

E. Antonio Chiocca
Harvard Medical School

Choi-Fong Cho
Brigham and Women's
   Hospital, Harvard Medical
   School

Jennifer Cosenza
Feinstein Kean Healthcare

Johnny Croy
Eli Lilly and Company

Kangwen Deng
AbbVie Inc.

Dario Doller
Sage Therapeutics

Xavier du Maine
Harvard Medical School

Lee Dudka
Dudka & Associates

Martin A. Duenas
Leidos

Suzanne Edavettal
Janssen Research &
   Development, LLC

Emmeline Edwards
National Center for
  Complementary and
  Integrative Health

Adam Fleisher
Eli Lilly and Company

Thomas Forbes
Children's National Health
  System

Peter Frinking
Bracco

Allyson Gage
Cohen Veterans Bioscience

Lei Gao
AbbVie Inc.

Hugo Geerts
In Silico Biosciences

Reza Ghodssi
University of Maryland

Alexandra Golby
Harvard Medical School,
  Brigham and Women's
  Hospital, Department of
  Neurosurgery

Marjorie Gondre-Lewis
Howard University College of
  Medicine

Viviana Gradinaru
California Institute of
Technology

Robert Greely
Biogen

Shenita-Ann Grymes
BrittNelle Health Services
  Group, LLC

Chenghua Gu
Harvard Medical School

Sean Han
Amgen

Joseph Hanig
Food and Drug
  Administration

Richard Hatzfeld
Feinstein Kean Healthcare, an
  Ogilvy Company

Ramona Hicks
One Mind

Stuart Hoffman
Office of Research and
  Development, Department
  of Veterans Affairs

Douglas Hunt
ArmaGen

Steven Hyman
Stanley Center for Psychiatric
  Research

Michael Irizarry
Eli Lilly and Company

Tom Jacobs
University of Texas

Brett Janosky
Amgen

Dominique Jennings
Celgene

Sophia Jeon
National Institute of
  Neurological Disorders and
  Stroke

Alexander Kabanov
Center for Nanotechnology in
  Drug Delivery, UNC
  Eshelman School of
  Pharmacy

Claire Kaplan
University of Maryland
  College Park

Kristin Kemmerich
National Research Council of
  Canada

Alireza Khaligh
University of Maryland

Sooja Kim
American Institute for Cancer
  Research

James Koenig
National Institute of
  Neurological Disorders and
  Stroke

Vinod Kulkarni
National Institute of
  Neurological Disorders and
  Stroke

Story Landis
National Institute of
  Neurological Disorders and
  Stroke (Emeritus)

Gerhard Leinenga
The University of Queensland

Na Li
Amgen

Sarah H. Lisanby
National Institute of Mental
  Health

Roger Little
National Institute on Drug
  Abuse

Linda Loyd
Ippfast Inc.

Lucy Lu
Merck

Yifeng Lu
AbbVie Inc.

Linda MacArthur
Center for Scientific Review,
  National Institutes of Health

Mary MacDonald
Engility

Husseini Manji
Janssen Research &
    Development, LLC

Timothy Mason
Law Office of Sylvia Chin-
    Caplan, LLC

Bill McCarty
Amgen

Michael McCaughan
Prevision Policy

David McMullen

Douglas Meinecke
National Institute of Mental
    Health

David Michelson
Merck

Laura Mitic
University of California, San
    Francisco Memory and
    Aging Center

Roscoe M. Moore, Jr.
PH RockWood LLC

Radha Murthy
Nimhans

Dylan Neel
Harvard University

Jorge L. Nina Espinosa
University of Puerto Rico

Bob Nocco
Chevron Corporation

Vicente Nunez
Harvard University

Colin O'Carroll
Ardmore Biotech Consulting

Sarah O'Connor
Amgen

Hie Page

Iason Papademetriou
Boston University

William Pardridge
University of California, Los
    Angeles

Taeeun Park
Harvard University

Cinthia Pastuskovas
Amgen

Mitesh Patel
Amgen

Nikunj Patel
Food and Drug
    Administration

Vikram Patel
Food and Drug
    Administration

Michele Pearson
National Institute of Mental
  Health

Nathalia Peixoto
George Mason University

Creighton Phelps
Retired, National Institute on
  Aging

Roger Phillips
Private consulting practice

Elizabeth Pimentel
Maryland University of
  Integrative Health

Andrea Pirzkall
Beigene

David Polidori
Janssen Research &
  Development, LLC

William Potter
National Institute of Mental
  Health

Darwin Prockop
Texas A&M University

Ipolia Ramadan
National Institutes of Health

Deepa Rao
Food and Drug
  Administration

Carolina Remos
Northwell Health

Carl Rhodes
Alexander and Associates

Max Robinowitz
Retired, Food and Drug
  Administration

Bob Roehr
Scientific American

Madelaine Romero

Hector Rosas-Hernandez
National Center for
  Toxicological Research

Susan Rosenbaum
Lauren Sciences LLC

Erik Runko
National Science Foundation

Lynn Rutkowski
Ossianix, Inc.

Ramkrishna Sadhukhan
AbbVie Inc.

Shilpa Sambashivan
Amgen

Ahmed Samir
Charite Berlin

Eric Schaeffer
Janssen Research &
  Development, LLC

Eugenia Schenecker
The George Washington
  University

Oliver Schmidt
Eli Lilly and Company

Ralf Seip
Sonacare Medical

Masha Sergeeva
DMPK4BIOTECH

Lisa Shafer
Teva Pharmaceuticals

Dhavalkumar Shah
University of New York at
  Buffalo, Department of
  Pharmaceutical Sciences

Lily Silayeva
Defense Threat Reduction
Agency

Len Singer
Smarterage LLC

Sanjaya Singh
Janssen Pharmaceutical
  Companies of Johnson &
  Johnson

Patroula Smpokou
Department of Health and
  Human Services

Krystyna Solarana
Food and Drug
  Administration

Andrew Sostek
Katanya

Barry Springer
Janssen Research &
  Development, LLC

Stinivasa Srinivasa
National Institute of Mental
  Health and Neuro-Sciences,
  Bangalore, India

Danica Stanimirovic
National Research Council of
  Canada

Pawel Stocki
Ossianix, Inc.

Bernd Stowasser
Sanofi

Jennifer Stratton
Teva Pharmaceuticals

Ron Swanson
Janssen Research &
  Development, LLC

Edmund Talley
National Institute of
  Neurological Disorders and
  Stroke/BRAIN Initiative

Amir Tamiz
National Institute of
  Neurological Disorders and
  Stroke

Ben Tang
Amgen

Hiroaki Tani
Eli Lilly and Company

Lorin Thompson
Fulcrum Therapeutics

Robert Thorne
University of Wisconsin–
  Madison

Jason Tien
Teva Pharmaceuticals

Kelsie Timbie
Focused Ultrasound
  Foundation

Wendy Toler
Consultant, Medical
  Affairs/Clinical
  Development

Alan Trachtenberg
Food and Drug
  Administration

Kathleen Tusaie
William Beckett & Associates

Rebecca Voelker
*Journal of the American
  Medical Association*

Meredith Wadman
Science magazine

Owen Wallace
Fulcrum Therapeutics

Frank Walsh
Ossianix, Inc.

Kuan Wang
Taipei Medical University

Lily Wang
Maimonides Cancer Center

Alex Watters
Wyss Institute

Andrew Welchman
The Wellcome Trust

Cole Werble
Prevision Policy, LLC

Matthew Whittaker
Food and Drug
  Administration

Krzysztof Wicher
Ossianix, Inc.

Dionna Williams
Johns Hopkins University

Dan Wolak
Amgen

Winifred Wu
Strategic Regulatory Partners,
  LLC

Shuyan Yi
Amgen

Nathan Yoganathan
KalGene Pharmaceuticals Inc.

Claudia Zamora
Zamora Consulting Group

Mark Zervas
Amgen

Berislav Zlokovic
University of Southern
  California